STOP STARTING OVER

STOP STARTING OVER

TRANSFORM YOUR FITNESS BY MASTERING YOUR PSYCHOLOGY

DEVAN KLINE

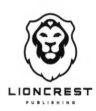

LIONCREST
PUBLISHING

STOP STARTING OVER

Transform Your Fitness by Mastering Your Psychology

ISBN   978-1-5445-1173-3 *Paperback*

978-1-5445-1172-6 *Ebook*

I dedicate this book to the women of Huntersville, North Carolina. You've given me the opportunity to live my dream and inspire lasting change all over the world. I couldn't have done this without your trust in me. I'll be forever grateful to you, and you'll never fully realize the positive effects you've had on my life.

CONTENTS

INTRODUCTION...9

1. STOP STARTING OVER................................27

2. DESIGNING YOUR LIFE..............................35

3. VISUALIZE YOUR "PERFECT DAY".........................49

4. CREATING LASTING CHANGE...............................55

5. WHEN WOULD "NOW" BE A GOOD TIME?...........67

6. THE PRINCIPLES OF MENTAL MASTERY...............83

7. THE PRINCIPLES OF EMOTIONAL MASTERY.......117

8. PRINCIPLES OF PHYSICAL MASTERY.................137

9. NUTRITION...163

10. RECOVERY...193

11. THE PRINCIPLES OF SPIRITUAL MASTERY.........201

12. OVERCOMING OBJECTIONS..............................211

13. THE MAGIC OF MOMENTUM...............................231

14. LIFE IS A UNIVERSITY.................................245

15. 80 PERCENT OF HAPPINESS..............................253

16. DEVELOPING YOUR DAILY RITUALS.....................261

CONCLUSION...267

ABOUT THE AUTHOR..273

INTRODUCTION

THE WARM-UP

I'm not your average trainer, and this isn't your average fitness book. Since 2012, I've had the privilege of personally training 20,000 clients and have helped thousands more through my Burn Boot Camps all over the United States. I've encountered people with all types of personalities, behaviors, and fitness goals, and I've learned that most of us go through life repeatedly chasing after the same goals with little progress—we never *truly* figure out why momentary motivation seems to fade so quickly. Through my experiences, I've discovered the common behaviors that clearly separate successful people from unsuccessful ones. I've developed a philosophy based on these findings that will give you an opportunity to stop setting the same goals and falling short. The words "I'll start over on Monday" will never come out of your mouth again!

I do not claim to have a degree in psychology, but observations of human behavior have molded me into a practical "fitness psychologist." After working with so many folks, I'd have to be an idiot not to notice the patterns that dictate success. I've been able to help clients achieve incredible results by uniting the study of human psychology with real, actionable steps that people can understand.

As a society, we've got fitness all wrong. Fitness isn't just about physical activity and getting a six-pack. Our mission should far transcend superficial selfies and dramatic weight loss programs. My life's journey is to help you and your loved ones create *lasting change* and never have to "start over" again.

In its current state, the fitness industry is grossly failing you. Despite fitness being available on every corner and all over social media, we are larger than ever. Nearly 70 percent of our country is overweight, 35 percent of adults are considered obese, and nearly 20 percent of children are overweight.[*] Those statistics should make it no surprise to you that only 17 percent of people have a gym membership.

These disturbing facts fuel my desire to give every ounce of energy to create lasting change, one family at a time.

---

[*]   "Obesity Rates & Trends Overview," *The State of Obesity*, https://stateofobesity.org/obesity-rates-trends-overview.

My goal is for this book to be the last one you'll ever need to design a healthy life for yourself and your loved ones.

We'll never create lasting change if we don't do something drastic. There must be a societal paradigm shift. For years, we've been obsessed with the newest diet plan, the latest workout fad, and the most innovative technology. We think that magic potions and popping pills are the cure-all, when the fact is, they don't work. Expecting them to create lasting change is like placing a Band-Aid over a gunshot wound. The bleeding stops momentarily, but you'll need a truckload of Band-Aids and an extremely high pain tolerance. Trends may work for thirty days, but they simply cannot sustain lasting results.

Everyone understands on an intellectual level that eating well and exercising often are what we *need* to do to be healthy. The problem is, we don't *want* to do it. If you Google "how to be healthy," you'll see 410 million results pop up, and it's obvious we aren't lacking in strategy. What we lack is purpose. We are missing an enchanting reason to look beyond the hurdles of today, hardships of tomorrow, and challenges of next year. It's time to create a long-term resolve founded on purpose and to drop the short-term focus of looking better. *That's* what will give you the clarity, strength, and follow-through to overcome all adversity on your journey.

Fitness is much more than working out three to six times

per week. It's an integration of physical, mental, emotional, and spiritual strength that stands on a foundation of psychological principles that govern your actions. When you find a purpose greater than "looking good," you'll never have to "start over" again.

THE STORY: 84 PLEASANT AVE.

Before we dive into our coaching, I want to share my story to give you context as to *how* I ended up pouring my heart out through this pen. I never had anyone "show me the way." Much of my philosophy was derived from necessity.

As a child, I never imagined I would be CEO of a fitness empire and an internationally recognized personal trainer. I was born in 1987, in Battle Creek, Michigan. I grew up in a low-income area; some might even call it the ghetto. My father was a part-time electrician, and my mom was a waitress at a local dive bar. They were both full-time alcoholics and drug abusers.

Their lifestyle revolved around partying, and that often led to physical violence in our home. The Battle Creek police frequented my home at 84 Pleasant Ave., which turned out to be not-so-pleasant, after all. I vividly remember all-out brawls between my parents that would leave my mom with black eyes, my dad covered in scratch marks, and our phone cords ripped out of the wall.

My parents weren't just violent with each other; they were also violent toward me and my siblings—a good share of blood was spilled in my childhood home. Being pushed down the stairs and having my head shoved through drywall by my father were regular occurrences. I tried to avoid the violence at all costs, but there was no getting around it in such a small home.

Eventually, my parents split up, and my mother forced my brother and me to accompany her while she chased boyfriends across the country. We had lived in six different states by the time I was in fifth grade. I can't say life would have been much better in Battle Creek, as my father was in and out of jail for drunk driving and domestic abuse of his new "flavor of the week." Eventually, my mother carted us back to Battle Creek to reunite with my father, as if she believed something would change, but nothing did. Our family dynamics picked up right where they left off.

My dad was a great athlete in his glory days, and his acceptance of me was dependent upon my athletic performance. When I was a sophomore in high school, I played on the varsity basketball team, and he berated me the first time I failed to score double digits in a game. He was drunk when I got home from the game that night. He made me shovel three feet of accumulated snow in our driveway, and when the task was done, I had to shoot one hundred baskets. He pushed me around and verbally abused me the entire time—I wasn't allowed to go inside until I made all the shots. It wasn't the best coaching tactic, but it pushed me to become a better athlete.

The lack of a childhood role model forced me to mature at a young age, and I used sports as a vehicle to develop physical, mental, emotional, and spiritual rituals. I was never the most talented athlete, but I played at a high level because I worked hard and put in long hours of practice. I knew there was a seventy-thirty chance of getting beat up or verbally abused at home, and that probability kept me on the field, on the court, or in the weight room.

THE TURNING POINT

My chaotic life spilled into my early high school years. My parents never got up early in the morning, so I made the long trek to school each day by foot. Eventually, I grew tired of the walk and solicited rides from friends. When I turned sixteen, I decided to buy myself a car. I worked my ass off for two consecutive summers to save $2,500 and buy a run-down 1999 Pontiac Grand Am. Only one headlight worked, and I had to jumpstart it during the cold Michigan winters, but I was very proud of it. Then, it was taken from me—by my mother. While I was away at a baseball tournament, she decided to flee town again. She stole my car, sold it, and used the money to move herself and my brother to Arizona. It was heartbreaking, and as I grappled with my emotions, something new was ignited in me. I'd had enough, and decided I never wanted to live the life of my parents.

Shortly after I made that decision, I found a Tony Robbins CD called *Personal Power* in my parents' old collection. Since I no longer had a car, I listened to it on my Sony Walkman during the long bike ride to school every day. I came to realize Tony was the role model I needed. His message made me believe, for the first time ever, that there was a greater experience of life beyond Battle Creek.

I came to realize that I didn't choose to be in my current situation—I was placed there. I couldn't control external circumstances, other people, their choices, and their judgments of me. But there were aspects of life I *could* control: my thoughts, my emotions, and the meaning I chose to give to the events in my life. I set out on a mission to take control of my circumstances and become the person God intended me to be. I became obsessed with studying psychology and began reading every sports-psychology book I could get my hands on.

MY SAVING GRACE

Through all of my childhood turmoil, I was blessed to have a rock, a person I could count on. Her name was Morgan, and she was my saving grace. We met when we were twelve, and it was instant puppy love. We spent our teenage years together, and her belief in me is a large part of why I am writing this book today.

Morgan encouraged me, kept me grounded, and helped me through tough times. When I wanted to quit or run away, she brought me back with purpose—she gave me something to look forward to. Her parents, Lorrie and Larry, were phenomenal and often saved me from my violent environment. Her mom let me stay the night (in an age-appropriate manner, of course), because she knew how difficult things were for me at home.

I continued to use the field and court as an escape from my troubled home life, and with support from Morgan, her family, my oldest brother Jason, and his wife Aubrey, I excelled in sports. My hard work came to fruition when I was seventeen and received an offer to play at Central Michigan University on a baseball scholarship. It was a breakthrough that overwhelmed my senses, my emotions, and my body. I remember feeling like I had made it to the top of the world! It was more than my ticket out of Battle Creek; it was an opportunity to do something extraordinary with my life, and I was determined to take full advantage of it.

The summer before college, the entrepreneur in me was born. I was sick of being broke, so I worked roofing jobs with my uncle. I saved enough money to buy another car, a 1989 Ford Probe. I immediately tuned up the car and flipped it on eBay. I used the earnings to buy another Pontiac Grand Am and repeated the process. I flipped four more cars over the next six months, until I was riding in a 2004 Ford Mustang and had about $5,000 to my name! As I approached my freshman year of college, my focus shifted from making money to playing baseball.

I went to Central Michigan University while Morgan attended Western Michigan, and we continued to date throughout college. I was a standout on the baseball team, and I received an offer to play for the San Francisco Giants. I was obsessively focused on becoming an MLB pitcher, so my entrepreneurial dreams were put on hold. Morgan and baseball were my life, but my big-league dreams were crushed when I was released from the organization after three seasons.

My Plan A—playing ball—had failed, and I felt lost. I never believed in creating a Plan B, so I had nowhere to turn. I believed it was weak to have a Plan B, because it created uncertainty in Plan A. I knew my relentless pursuit of my goals had landed me the Central Michigan scholarship and the Giants contract. I chose to be certain that same work ethic would lead me to a new calling—a new purpose in life.

FINDING MY TRUE PURPOSE

The time I spent practicing and playing sports led me to fall in love with fitness and nutrition. I traveled for six years while playing for Central Michigan and the Giants, and I stayed with various host families in different cities. I'd assumed that many families experienced the "Kline dynamics," but I couldn't have been more wrong—I got a taste of "normal" family issues. My host families were encouraging, caring, and loving but still struggled with unhappiness, similarly to my parents. They didn't turn to drugs and alcohol but rather to food, physical laziness, and an abundance of excuses to combat life's problems. This created a lack of vitality and energy that only seemed to contribute to those feelings of unhappiness.

When I was released from the Giants, I remember sitting in a hotel room in Scottsdale, Arizona, and bawling my eyes out. My dream was suddenly over, and I had no idea what to do with myself. The one person I could call for advice was Morgan, and she reminded me how proud I should be of my accomplishments. She said,

"DEVAN, LOOK HOW FAR YOU'VE COME. JUST KEEP MOVING FORWARD."

I remember mentally repeating the phrase "keep moving" as I boarded a plane to reunite with her in Naples, Florida.

During my flight home, I had my breakthrough moment. You know those "ah-ha" moments when you feel like a light bulb turns on? Yes, it was one of those. I recalled the satisfaction I experienced when teaching my host families the principles I used to maintain control of my life while growing up. My presence in their homes created an apparent contagious energy as I felt my positivity as well as nutrition and fitness knowledge rub off on them.

My greater purpose was clear. I made it my mission to positively impact as many people as I could, and a few months later, I created a fitness program that was inspired by my host families. My early years of studying fitness, nutrition, and psychology allowed me to pay it forward at a young age, and I found pure satisfaction in helping other people. It was a fulfillment I had never experienced in baseball, and I fell in love with it!

Thus, my first program was born, "Lightning 900." I trained women in Southwest Florida to "Burn 900 Calories Lightning Fast," while teaching them to put themselves first for a change. I found my energy and presence to be more contagious than ever. My program caught fire, and within ninety days, I was one of the most recognized trainers in Southwest Florida.

My training career was just taking off when Morgan was offered an advancement opportunity with her company.

If she accepted, she would have to relocate to Charlotte, North Carolina. She deserved this promotion, and I would support her, because she had supported me my entire life. I knew that I would be at home wherever I was, as long as she was with me.

THE QUEEN CITY

Morgan moved, and I stayed behind in Naples for a few months to finish out my personal training contracts. I worked for twelve hours at the gym and spent the following five waking hours creating what is now known as Burn Boot Camp. I used those months to put one of my favorite Tony Robbins quotes into practice: "Success is not about your resources. It's about how resourceful you are with what you have."

When I wasn't training clients, I studied marketing, gym operations, HTML coding, video editing, legal issues, finance, and business operations. Within three months, I had created a brand and a website, and I'd pieced together the legal, financial, and operational elements of a business using the only resource I had: Google. I learned all I needed to know to run a business, and I was ready for the move. Now, my only problem was figuring out how to start a business with no money.

When I arrived in Charlotte, I spent thirty days researching cheap options for a boot camp location. I had no financial history, and after being turned down for several commercial leases, I felt stuck. Again, being resourceful, I subleased a gymnastics center and its parking lot, and I ran the first Burn Boot Camp session on April 19, 2012.

THE PARKING LOT DAYS

After the big move, I only had $600 left of my Lightning 900 earnings, and I used the last dollar I had to buy dumbbells and exercise mats. I had zero dollars in my advertising budget, so I got my first clients by visiting a local supermarket. I gave T-shirts to women who looked like they were into fitness, and I offered them a free thirty-day trial. I still have no idea how such a "compelling offer" to work out in a dark parking lot at 5 a.m. with a complete stranger actually worked!

Twenty-one women signed up for the first Burn Boot Camp sessions, and ten showed for the first three. I got "no-showed" the last two days of the first week, so I had a decision to make. I recalled my car-flipping days and decided being broke wasn't an option. I discovered the root cause of my problem was that I was the best-kept secret in town! At that moment, I dedicated my business to being a marketing company. The product was Burn Boot Camp, and I began my deep dive into social media, public relations, and content creation. I even reached out to a reporter, and she wrote a story about my journey in the local paper. My parking lot was flooded with clients the next week!

Positive momentum soon followed, and more people began to show up. The boot camp grew from zero paying clients to 250 paying clients within six months. I felt like I had made it! With $18,000 in my bank account, I had room to breathe and could finally support the woman who had supported me my entire life. It was the most satisfying feeling, and I will never forget the moment when Morgan decided to quit her corporate job and pursue her dream alongside me. We got engaged and began our lives as the founders of Burn Boot Camp.

GROWTH AND REWARD

Supporting Morgan was only part of the reward for my hard work. From the beginning, I wanted to help women, especially mothers, break free from their limiting beliefs. I wanted everyone to realize that fitness transcends simply working out. I grew increasingly curious regarding why people like me who grew up with nothing could live happily, while those with far more to be proud of were often dissatisfied. I began keenly studying human behavior and recording my findings in a daily journal. I had a desire to expand the positive impact, so we started three more "parking lot" boot camps and hired other trainers to lead them.

I thought I was at the peak of success when two trainers contacted me and asked how they could bring Burn Boot Camp to their cities—Morgan and I had never considered this type of expansion as a possibility. I went to an attorney for a licensing agreement, and soon after, Burn Boot Camp had seven locations. By the end of the year, each location had its own brick-and-mortar facility—we had experienced rapid growth and could no longer split space and schedules with other businesses.

THE FRANCHISE OPPORTUNITY

After our facilities were up and running in 2014, a man named Jeff Dudan became my landlord. We grew to be friends, and one day he said in these exact words, "Dude, your business model is sexy. Have you ever thought about franchising?" He had a playful smile on his face. Jeff is a seasoned franchisor and was the first person to see potential in a nationwide push for Burn Boot Camp. His instincts were right. If I wanted to expand my reach, I couldn't do it alone. I needed help from people who shared my philosophy: make an impact that could change people's lives forever.

Usually, it takes eight to twelve months to get a franchise going, but I approached the endeavor with a laser focus, and we were ready to go in three months. I was told success would be three locations the first year. I established ten locations in the first week, and we continued to experience explosive growth from that point forward. Since our debut on February 19, 2015, Burn Boot Camp has been one of the fastest-growing franchises in the world, with plans for 15,000 locations worldwide. We turned our dreams into goals, and our goals into reality.

I've personally worked with 20,000 clients over the past five years, and I've mentored hundreds of trainers who have impacted hundreds of thousands more. I'm fully committed to my clients, franchise partners, trainers, and followers—this mission has always been about them. And right now, it's all about you, the reader.

FINDING THE MISSING PIECE

Achieving your desired fitness level is 90 percent psychology and 10 percent strategy. Your mindset (that 90 percent) ultimately determines success, but so many of us begin with that 10 percent, the "how to," rather than developing a compelling purpose.

For example, imagine we are in a room with 1,000 people, and I ask everyone to raise their hand if they believe eating healthily and exercising often are good strategies to become fit. How many hands do you think would shoot into the sky? If you guessed all of them, you're right! If that's true and everyone knows it, then why is

70 percent of the American population struggling with weight? What is the missing dynamic here? If everyone cognitively understands this strategy to be true, then why isn't everyone fit and healthy? It's because there is a fundamental flaw we collectively share: we place far too much focus on the "how to." We know what we need to do to be healthy, but it's obvious that the majority of us aren't doing it.

By this example, we see that knowledge is not power—it only holds *potential* power. Your cognitive understanding doesn't hold enough juice to move you to action. The real power is in mastering the art of taking action, but relying on that alone isn't a sound strategy, either. People don't develop routines and rituals based on even the strongest desire to execute strategies. There has to be something more. I've made it my life's mission to use my studies and my own personal resolve to fill in the gaps—and help you identify the missing pieces.

During the early days of my career, I knew that in order to impact health communities all around the world, I needed to find the answer to the fundamental question: "what's missing?"

Then I had another "ah-ha" moment. People generally don't realize the power of their minds. So many of us are obsessed with which gym to attend, which shoes to wear, and which foods to eat that we fail to ask ourselves the following two questions:

"What do I want out of my life?" Or, in other words, "What is my desired outcome?"

"Why do I want it?" Or, in other words, "What is my purpose?"

After realizing the importance of these questions, "Focus Meetings" were born. When I first meet with clients, they expect to have a fitness or nutrition consultation. We don't. Instead, we dig into their psychology and work to get their minds right. We start with the 90 percent—the psychology—and *then* figure out the strategy once we've determined an outcome and purpose.

Developing a meal or exercise plan won't change your life. It's time to get to the root cause of the obesity problem: our personal psychological makeup. One thing I've learned from experience is that you'll become what you think about most often. So, continue reading if you're ready to reprogram your psychology, install new belief systems, and stop starting over!

★ CHAPTER 1 ★

STOP STARTING OVER

How many times have you tried to lose weight and failed? Or lost weight only to gain it back? How many times have you said, "I'm done eating like a pig! I'm going to eat healthily from now on," only to revert to old habits a few days or weeks later? I want you to stop starting over. I want you to be done with New Year's resolutions. I will help you download a new philosophy into your mind so that you can make constant, consistent progress. Picking up this book is the first step toward creating positive changes in your life, and I'll guide you in this process by leading with practical psychology. As we dive into this book, you'll see that strategies are the least of our concern. As I mentioned earlier, this isn't your average fitness book, so if you're expecting another cookie-cutter diet or short-term exercise plan, set this down and head to Google for your answers.

Health and fitness professionals often tell us how many calories to eat per day, how much sleep we need, and which workout routines yield the best results. However, every human being is different—every person has different needs. While fuel, recovery, and movement are consistently necessary, the proper ratios of each will differ with each individual and their goals.

My goal is to give you the opportunity to think for yourself. This book will cause you to question what you believe to be your reality and open your mind to your actuality. I cannot make decisions for you, but I'll provide you with the framework to make choices. The plan will be all yours, so you can be true to yourself. We'll develop a brand-new mindset and create absolute certainty that you can maximize your quality of life by following a plan—one on your terms that you can stick with for the long haul.

REDEFINING YOUR STANDARDS

If you asked me for one piece of coaching advice to take your life to the next level, I would say: *raise your standards.* I know what you're thinking: "Thank you, Devan, for the deep, thought-provoking advice," as you roll your eyes. This statement is simple, yet so powerful. It's hard to believe it can have any impact, because humans tend to gravitate toward complicated philosophy and shy away from simplicity. I suppose we assume that since life is already hard, changing it must be even harder.

AS SURE AS THE SUN RISES EACH MORNING, YOU HAVE THE OPPORTUNITY TO REDEFINE WHO YOU ARE AND WHAT YOU CAN BECOME EACH DAY.

This is a simple choice you must make for yourself. You can continue to be numb to your past, not question why you think the way you do, and carry on with life, convincing yourself that your situation "is what it is." Or, you can forget that bullshit and pick up what I'm putting down.

THE ORIGIN OF YOUR STANDARDS

Have you ever questioned why you are the way you are? When did you become a sugar addict? When did you define yourself as "not a fitness person"? When did you decide you weren't smart enough? Sexy enough? Talented enough?

Chances are, these thoughts come from past conditioning. As children, we could do *anything*, and somewhere along the way, your environment conditioned you to think differently. Most likely your parents, friends, or other family members convinced you that you're not good enough. They never did this maliciously, and their intentions were to protect you from pain, but it does no good to continue through life without questioning where your standards come from. After all, experiencing pain in your life is necessary to grow as a human being.

Whose permission are you waiting for to live the life you want? Whose approval do you need to begin questioning your past? What's stopping you from changing the course of your life moving forward?

Standards are a choice. You either have poor, good, great, or outstanding standards for yourself, and right now, being brutally honest is the only way to begin the process of lasting change. Who set the standards for your life? Who dictated that this was the way it would be forever? Take a moment to consider your standards, because you'll always get exactly what you're willing to tolerate.

People with *poor standards* will experience a life of pain. A fast food diet, lack of exercise, bingeing on television, and being unhappy will result in a shorter life span. The people with these standards will minimize the quality of their lives. These are the standards of people who live to eat, not eat to live.

Those with *good standards* will get poor results. Have you ever heard someone say, "I'm good about working out, so why don't I see the results?" Or, "I'm a good husband. Why did my wife divorce me?" Or, "I am a good employee. Why did they let me go?" The answer is that good standards in today's society yield poor results. A good standard is one of contentment and complacency. "Good" just isn't going to cut it. There's a bounding leap to the next level of standards that separates those who are content from those who are motivated to live life at a higher level.

Individuals with *great standards* will get average results. These are the people who work their asses off to make ends meet. People with great standards will live an "okay" life, and there is nothing wrong with that. If this is you, then I want you to put this book down right now and continue being average; I can't help you excel if you don't want to help yourself. The next level of standards, outstanding standards, is only two millimeters away, but you've *really* got to want it.

I exist to serve those who have outstanding standards or who desire to be outstanding human beings. These are the people who are willing to get up at 5 a.m. to work out if they have to. These are the ones who want to succeed so badly that they are willing to commit to anything—and who strive for happiness and progression each day. These are the people who have committed to living life at the highest possible level, and want to reach physical, mental, emotional, and spiritual mastery.

So, what standards do you have for yourself? I cannot

answer this question for you, but if you want more out of life, you're in the right place. I will be hard on you during our time together, but that's why you picked up this book in the first place. If you're still reading, then I know you are ready to take your life to an outstanding place.

THE DECISION TO BE OUTSTANDING

If you feel you're in a bad place right now, this book will rock your world. If you're in an awesome place, this book will show you the next level! It's for anyone who desires to reach their maximum potential. My promise to you is that this book will be an inspiration and will help you create strategies to reach your goals by installing new belief systems, truly in the sense of *reprogramming* your brain. I've developed the philosophy within this book over the past fifteen years of my life, and it has helped countless people already. It's now *your* time to choose if you will be the next one to adopt an outstanding standard for yourself and commit to excellence.

This book is not for people who wish to be mediocre or for those who are comfortable being comfortable. It's for those who are experiencing discomfort or pain and realize the pain of remaining the same is greater than the pain of change. This book is for people who are ready to take it to the next level—those who are hungry for more.

If you aren't hungry for change in your life, then put this book down now, because you won't benefit from it. But if you're ready to be challenged from a place of love and support, turn the page and begin designing the life you deserve.

★ CHAPTER 2 ★

DESIGNING YOUR LIFE

DISCOVERING YOUR NORTH STAR

Have you ever wondered what the difference is between people who seem to succeed at everything vs. those who fail and give up? This question is the foundation of my life's work. I've spent years asking probing questions of real clients who've struggled with constantly starting over, and I've finally found the answer.

It's simple. Successful people know exactly what they want and why they want it, and they spend every waking moment attacking their goals. Those who achieve at the highest level have a clearly defined purpose. As my teacher Tony Robbins says, "Clarity is power." They've discovered an enchanting purpose and view success as the only option. They believe in a force so strong that they literally become unstoppable human beings. There's no obstacle, external event, or excuse that is powerful enough to derail the actions that will lead them to their ultimate desire. They don't always know *how* to get there, but they adopt a belief that accomplishes the goal mentally and emotionally prior to the physical manifestation.

Those who repeatedly "start over" wander through life never truly understanding their purpose. They think life is happening *to* them, not *for* them. They set goals aimlessly without conviction, which leaves them uncertain as to whether or not they will achieve the goal. Their motivation only lasts for a few weeks, and then they revert back to old habits. There's no clearly defined purpose that pulls them through times of adversity. Why does this happen? Most often, it's because they are too focused on the strategy.

Do the following questions sound familiar to you? Which gym should I join? Which clothes should I wear? What's the best diet plan? How many times per week should I work out? Should I lift weights or do cardio? How many calories should I eat? The answers to these questions won't matter unless you find your desired outcome and purpose first.

Whether you're crushing life at the moment or are at rock bottom, I want to challenge you to clearly define two things: your outcome and your purpose. I've demanded this from my clients, and the majority of them couldn't give me a clearly defined answer. This led me to understand that most of us never ask these questions of ourselves. When you can answer them with your heart, you will have the foundation for a journey of unlimited success.

What do you really want to transform?

Why do you really want to transform?

I call the answers to these questions the "North Star," and they will become the guiding light for every decision you make. Creating lasting change in your health boils down to two things: pain and pleasure. The pain of not reaching your goals must be far greater than the pain of getting up at 5 a.m. to work out, making a healthy choice at dinner, or heading to the gym after a long day of work. The only way to create this projection of pain is to answer these questions.

I want you to take some time right now to discover your North Star. After you read this chapter, get out a piece of paper and get to work. Emotion creates motion. Your answers will establish an emotional connection to what you care about most, cutting off any possibility, story, or excuse you've used in the past. By connecting strongly with your North Star, you'll start to think and act in ways that drive you to success.

INSTRUCTIONS

Get out a piece of paper, a pen, and a stopwatch. Set a timer for fifteen minutes when answering each one, for a total of thirty minutes. I understand you're a busy person and this will be a time commitment, but I'm asking you this: Are you willing to spend thirty minutes to change the course of your entire life? Is it worth it to you? The most successful people in the world have taken the time to thoroughly answer these questions to understand the outcomes they will produce. To achieve your fitness goals (or any goal in life) you *must* know these answers. Without them, lasting change is impossible.

Please spend thirty consecutive, uninterrupted minutes with this exercise. Don't break up the question/answer sessions into separate segments. Don't play music in the background, cook dinner, or have kids grabbing your legs. Find a place of solitude, and take thirty minutes to gain clarity and control of your life.

Be Specific

Motivational speaker and author Brian Tracy likens our minds to buckets of dirty water. When there is dirt mixed in a bucket of water, it appears murky. It takes a while for the dirt to settle at the bottom, but when it does, we see a distinct separation between the dirt and the water.

It's important to spend thirty minutes answering these questions so that the dirt has time to settle and your mind is clear. Working on each question for fifteen minutes also forces you to get deep into your thoughts.

The first six to ten minutes of this exercise will be a breeze, but once you get past this time frame, your mind may go blank. Keep thinking through this period. After a few more minutes, your mind will become clear—your brain will have had the chance to process what you're asking. You'll begin writing again, and you won't stop. There may be a few pauses lasting two or three minutes at a time, but you'll stay on track.

Be on the alert for generic answers. These are the types of answers produced by the brain, rather than your heart. If your first thought is, "I want to be fit," then welcome to the club. Everyone has that thought, and there's no specific emotional connection to your life if you simply want to be fit. If you sit for a bit longer, your answer will become more specific: "I want to be fit because I will feel confident, and my example will help my two-year-old grow up with confidence." That answer comes from your heart. The reason is specific to *you* and your life.

I want to emphasize that you cannot answer these questions in a state of frustration or fear. Ensure that you are in a peak state of mind. A great time for this exercise is immediately after physical activity, when endorphins and dopamine have you feeling happy and proud.

Keep reading, and you'll find a set of "thought starters" that I'll use to get your juices flowing. As you're answering these questions, I want you to *feel* them. Remember: motion is created by emotion, so take the time to visualize how your answers make you feel before writing them.

WHAT DO YOU REALLY WANT TO TRANSFORM?

This question is about your outcome. The answers to this question should be all about you and how achieving your goals will make you feel. How do you want to feel about your loved ones? How do you want to feel about your coworkers and friends? What do you want to be proud of? How do you want to be portrayed as a professional? Where do you want to live? What do you want to have? What type of friendships do you want to cultivate? What type of financial freedom is in your life? What's your relationship with God (or a higher power) like? How do you feel about yourself? What kind of discipline do you want to create?

WHY DO YOU REALLY WANT TO TRANSFORM?

This question is about your purpose, or, in other words, how achieving your goals will impact other people. Who loves you the most? Why is this goal important to your loved ones? Why do you want this for them? What do you want your significant other to think about you? Why is this important to them? What do you want your coworkers to say about you? How does your freedom impact others? How does your goal impact your relationship with God (or your higher power)? How do you want your parents to feel about you?

BE OUTRAGEOUS

Take thirty minutes to write down everything you want, even if something feels ridiculous. It doesn't matter if your goals seem outrageous to you right now! The people who change the world are the ones who first change themselves, and that change often begins by setting ambitious, audacious goals.

When defining why you want this, trust your gut, and trust the process. Think of the people in your life who will be positively affected by these changes. How will it make you feel when they are affected? Finding the *why* consists of thinking about who you love the most and connecting those people to your purpose. The only way you create lasting change is by attaching your goals to something bigger than yourself.

How Will You Get There?

It doesn't matter. Overanalyzing strategy can be paralyzing. It's easy to get overwhelmed by all the information out there about losing weight and getting healthy. When you have no idea which direction to go, it's tempting to curl up into a ball and decide to stay put—you're fearful of making mistakes. The truth is, you don't have to know any of the strategies yet.

The Power of Love

Let's get deeper into the psychology of creating lasting change. You must connect the pain of *not* attaining your goals directly to a significant loss of love. Love is the oxygen of life, and we will go to great lengths mentally, emotionally, spiritually, and physically to protect the relationships and connections in our lives.

LIFE IS NOTHING WITHOUT LOVE.

What would you do if your mother or father became extremely ill, and the only way to save them was to come up with $25,000 to cover their medical expenses? Certainly, you'd find a way to raise the money. Initially, you'd have no clue where to start, but your love for them is so strong that *not* raising the money wouldn't be an option. How creative would you get? Wouldn't you go to great lengths to save them?

As human beings, we are capable of astounding things. There's nothing that is impossible. I despise the word "unbelievable," because I have witnessed amazing clients overcome their limiting beliefs, and I've proved it with my own story as well. There's nothing that is unbelievable to me. When a loss of love is on the line, you'll do whatever is necessary to maintain the connection.

Project the Pain

Throughout this book, I don't suggest that life is all sunshine and roses. You won't catch me giving a seminar, training clients, or having one-on-one meetings telling people to "be positive," and it will change their lives. Negativity and pain are powerful tools when used appropriately. I'm going to ask something of you that's pretty crazy, and this will be the first strategy I teach you to lock in your purpose.

You're reading this book because you're sick of starting over. The strategies you've tried thus far simply aren't meeting your expectations. To stop starting over, you must understand that trying the same strategy repeatedly but expecting different results is the literal definition of insanity. You're not an insane person, but failure to change your strategies will leave you stuck in the same place. So, are you willing to play this out with me and attempt something you've never tried before? If so, good. Keep reading.

When this exercise is done to completion, you will associate so much pain with *not* reaching your goals that your subconscious mind will default to behaviors that align with your North Star. This is an intense exercise, and it *only* works if you're truly committed to lasting change and fully playing it out. Initially, it will feel stupid, but I've helped save lives, bodies, marriages, and careers with this single exercise. Here we go!

I want you to vividly imagine the following. Don't just think about it—*feel it.*

Visualize dragging on your poor nutrition and fitness habits for five more years. Imagine how disgusting you feel about yourself. Look into a mirror and examine every inch of your body—the fat rolls and excess body fat. How disappointed are you in yourself? Imagine not being able to play with your children because you're too tired. How badly does that suck? Spend a few moments being disgusted with the state of your body. Notice how your face changes and how painful this feeling is.

Now, drag those bad habits out for ten years. After eating ten years of fast food and not moving your body, what happens to it? How disgusted are you now? How gross do you feel? Imagine having to buy brand new clothes, being ashamed to wear a swimsuit and embarrassed of yourself in public. Imagine your significant other walking out on you because you don't even love yourself any more. How painful is that feeling? Vividly imagine this, and feel yourself slipping away.

Now, take it twenty years out. What is your life like, if you are even alive? Imagine yourself in a fat, lazy, unmotivated body, sitting on the couch and barely able to move. Imagine yourself double the weight you are now. How does it feel to have a seatbelt extender on an airplane? How does it feel to walk around with a fat and swollen body? Feel the pain of everyone leaving you and living life alone, because you failed to love yourself enough to make a small series of changes years ago.

I want you to stop right now. Spend ten minutes visualizing this projected pain in your life. I know it sounds intense and harsh, but this is science at work. Our brains are 2 million years old and only have one job: to protect us from pain. When you neuro-associate (connect your mind to) pain and it *feels real*, your brain has no choice but to protect you. This isn't some bullshit strategy I've made up—this is hundreds of years of brain science being delivered to you in practical form.

Do this exercise every day for twenty-one days straight. Repeat the same questions, feel the same feelings, and let them intensify with each day. Imagine it so vividly that it becomes real to you. This will reprogram your mind and associate your projected behaviors with an extreme loss of love, which subconsciously forces you to change in order to protect that love.

MILLIONS OF STRATEGIES

You may not be ready for the "Projection of Pain" strategy yet, but I have found this to be the most universally beneficial strategy for clients who take it seriously. Some strategies in this book will work well for you, and others won't. Scrap the ones that don't work, and focus on the ones that do. What you *won't* do is try the same strategy over and over, hoping for a different result. If something doesn't work, you'll try something else. If that doesn't work, you'll try something else. If *that* doesn't work, what will you do? Try something else? Nailed it!

There are millions of strategies to try, and I promise you won't run out. As long as you have the conviction and belief that you will reach your North Star, it doesn't matter which strategy you choose. Connecting emotion and loss of love to your North Star generates the momentum for you to take control of your fitness—to stop starting over!

This is the last time you will need to create a plan to change your life. You've already changed it—consider it changed. It's been done inside of you, mentally and emotionally.

These are no longer dreams—they are goals. And now, it's time to make those goals a reality.

★ CHAPTER 3 ★

VISUALIZE YOUR "PERFECT DAY"

You have your North Star—the what and the why. If you skipped this exercise in the previous chapter, go back and do it right now. If you don't understand exactly what you want and why you want it, you'll just be going through the motions during the rest of this book.

When I first started my career and my family, I began to see how powerful visualization is. Every self-help guru and motivator on the planet talks about its importance. There's a reason the most successful people in the world all believe in visualizing—it's because it works!

Don't let yourself fall into the "familiarity trap." This happens when you hear principles so often that they become white noise and you don't buy into them. Success leaves clues, and if the smartest people in the world collectively agree visualization can change your life, I think you should give it a try!

Now that you understand the projection of pain and know how to create a neuro-association with the loss of love, we need to create a positive association with a pleasurable life full of love, laughter, and joy! Wherever there is pain, you need to fill it with pleasure to lock in lasting change!

CREATE YOUR "PERFECT LIFE"

People have two identities: the shell identity and the core identity. When we first meet someone, they usually say something like, "Hi, I'm Susan. I'm a banker at First National." They introduce themselves only at the shallow, surface level. This is their shell identity.

When I introduce myself, I don't say, "I'm Devan, and I'm the CEO of Burn Boot Camp." I introduce myself as my core person: "I'm a thirty-year-old father, husband, and entrepreneur. I'm driven by my family and positively impacting every life I touch."

You must make sure that your core identity and your North Star for your fitness goals appropriately align. For example, I've asked 20,000 clients what they really wanted from their transformation, and a percentage of them said they wanted to be bodybuilders. However, we completed internet copywriter Frank Kern's "Perfect Day" exercise as a visualization tactic, and bodybuilding was nowhere to be found. They were allowing external influences—like social media—trick them into trying to be someone else.

I'M A HUGE PROPONENT OF "DOING YOU."
BE DIFFERENT. BE WEIRD. BE *YOU*!

Letting your environment dictate who you are is disingenuous and will ultimately lead to unhappiness. My clients were fascinated by bodybuilders, but that wasn't the outcome they desired for their lives. Bodybuilders make sacrifices that I knew these clients were unwilling to make—it wasn't in their core identity.

Perhaps they'd never had the opportunity to truly identify who they were. Without knowing your true self, it's extremely difficult to navigate life. It's an uncomfortable conversation to have with yourself, and the truth is most of us go through life as our shell version—we never identify ourselves at the core level. I want to make this conversation extremely easy and fun for you. The Perfect Day exercise below will help define who you are at the core level and what you truly care about in life. Ultimately, this will dictate your daily actions.

THE PERFECT DAY EXERCISE

If you had to live one day over and over for the rest of your life, with no consequences or limitations, what would that day look like?

That question carries some weight, doesn't it? To lend a hand in answering it, I've developed a set of follow-up questions. Answer these on paper, in paragraph form. When you're done, the answer will reveal who you *really* are. The purpose of this exercise is to develop introspective confidence, and I suggest you cross-reference your North Star with your newfound, core identity. Do your "what" and "why" lead you to living this perfect day? If so, you're ready to keep moving forward! If not, you'll adjust your North Star, not your core identity.

As you're going through and forming your Perfect Day, think chronologically. Put your Perfect Day together, and be as specific as possible. The more detail you insert, the more clearly you'll identify your core self.

- ★ **What would you do first thing in the morning?** What time would you get up? Who would you be with? Where would you live?
- ★ **Who loves you, and who do you love?** How does this love make you feel? Who are you sharing your life with? What type of freedom do you have together?

- ★ **What activity is in your life?** What are your rituals? What do you do for fun? What car do you drive?
- ★ **What is your work life like?** Do you work? If you don't work outside the home, what do you do? What are you passionate about? How much time do you spend with family?

You might be asking how this exercise reveals who you truly are. We get one shot in this life, so if you had to repeat a single day over and over, you'd do the things you were extremely passionate about and spend time with those you love the most. You'd waste zero time and effort. When you know what this day looks like, you've identified yourself at the core level and put your values on paper. You don't do what society expects you to do but what *you* want to do; you focus on what *you* care about. The answers to these questions reveal who you are!

A CLEAR VISION OF YOUR PERFECT DAY

Now, I want you to spend every waking hour for the rest of your life working to obtain your Perfect Day. As long as it's aligned with the physical and quantum laws of the universe, you can achieve anything you desire. Your mind is the most powerful and complex element known to man, so it's time to open up new possibilities and master your psychology!

MOMS ARE ROCK STARS

I want to take a moment to address the mothers reading this book. If you think you are "just a mom," please know that you are so much more than that. You're a caregiver, nurturer, chef, entertainer, and educator—and the list goes on and on. You do so many things, and you excel at each one—there's no way to justify the thought that you are "just a mom." You're a rock star, and more!

When I started leading boot camp in a parking lot and said I was going to change the world, people thought I was crazy. The program started as a "Fit Community of Moms," because I noticed how prevalent the "just a mom" mentality was. My Huntersville, North Carolina, moms banded together to rid the community of this poisonous thought, and they are the reason millions of moms around the world are dropping the title "Just a Mom" for "Mom, the Rock Star!"

This is a shout out to them! Thank you, gals, for believing in yourselves and showing moms all over the world that they are the toughest, most talented, and most perseverant people on the planet. Together, we are changing the world! Who's crazy now?

CHAPTER 4

CREATING LASTING CHANGE

We don't want to create temporary changes. The goal of this book is to develop *lasting change*. You can reprogram your mind to believe that you can attract anything you want in life! There is no more starting over. There are no more New Year's resolutions to get fit. You'll never have to "diet down" for summer again. It's time to start living life on your own terms—I believe that's the definition of happiness. Do what you want, when you want, with whom you want. That is the power of lasting change that is created when you design your own life.

PUT YOUR MASK ON FIRST

We're wrong if we believe achieving fitness goals will make us happy. Our dreams and goals must transcend fitness and physical appearance. It's a huge mistake to think that pouring all of your available resources into your fitness transformation will create happiness. Putting equal emphasis on your mental, emotional, and spiritual makeup is essential to achieving ultimate transformation.

How many times have you heard the term "work/life balance"? It's used often, and I feel this term doesn't accurately describe what we all try to achieve. The very nature of a balance beam or scale is that when one side becomes heavier, the other becomes lighter, or in this case, less significant—both sides must be equal to create balance.

Is there an area of your life that weighs heavy on one side of the scale? If you're a mother, it's likely that the scale is heavy on the side of children and family, and there's minimal emphasis placed on your personal well-being. To achieve equality, something must be added or removed. You could begin to tip the scale in favor of fitness, thinking that will make you happy, but you'll just end up unbalanced once again. For that reason, Morgan and I have adopted a different philosophy. We call it *holistic integration.*

Many people—especially women and mothers—put everything and everyone else above themselves. Not taking care of ourselves has become a major societal problem, and I believe it's a root cause of the global obesity crisis.

Being selfish is viewed as taboo, but without being happy with you who are, how can you possibly create happiness for others?

YOU WILL NEVER GAIN AN ABUNDANCE OF LIFE, ENERGY, OR VITALITY IF YOU AREN'T YOUR OWN NUMBER ONE PRIORITY.

When your tank is constantly empty, you don't have enough fuel to give back to the other priorities in your life. Focusing on the needs of others before your own needs doesn't benefit you (or them) in any way. It drains your energy, and you become a tired parent, impassionate lover, and poor performer at work. What is so bad about being selfish, if it means practicing good nutrition, getting regular physiological stimulation, and regularly feeding your mind?

It's time to put yourself first, love yourself more, and fulfill your own needs so that you can give others your best. Burn Boot Camp was founded on this very philosophy. From working with clients, I've realized that it's extremely difficult to for human beings to understand this concept. Try to think of it this way. When we board an airplane, the flight attendant instructs us to put our own oxygen masks on before assisting others with theirs. If you don't have air to breathe, you can't help others, and you suck the air away from them as well. To properly care for yourself, you must make it a priority to attend to your mental, physical, emotional, and spiritual needs with deliberate intention.

THE SCIENCE BEHIND SELFLESSNESS

It's not just mentally counterintuitive for you to be selfish—your body's biochemistry also fights against it. The moment children are born, parents develop higher levels of oxytocin, a powerful hormone that acts as a neurotransmitter in the brain. This regulates social interaction and sexual reproduction, and it plays a huge role in behaviors such as mother-infant bonding, milk release, empathy, and generosity. From the time our children are born or we meet our significant other, the deck is stacked against us.

Luckily, God has blessed human beings to be the only creatures on the planet who can question their very existence. This power allows us to differentiate between right and wrong and to make decisions that are contrary to our biological makeup. We are unselfish by default, so you have to make the *decision* to be selfish.

LOVE IS OXYGEN

To me, family is everything and the reason I take care of myself. Probably much like you, the love for my family is deeply rooted in my North Star, and the way they feel about me is fuel that drives me forward. A family's overall spiritual, emotional, and mental health directly influences their physical health. As the leader of your family, it's your responsibility to ensure discipline in all these areas. How can you install discipline in your children that you don't have installed in yourself?

In order to influence your family, you must be influenced. In order to move your family, you must be moved. How can you dare expect your family to love, respect, and forgive themselves if you've never done it? You can't encourage them to chase their dreams if they've spent a lifetime watching you do the opposite.

I'm a father first, a husband second, and everything else comes after that. With that being said, the first thing on my mind every day is taking care of myself. I spend the majority of my time, fifteen hours a day, working on my businesses so that my children will never experience life the way I did. I work out and eat well so that I can come home with energy and spend two hours of quality time with them before they go to bed.

Now, do you see how being selfish is necessary to the happiness of your family?

I've noticed in my own life that when I am self-aware and take care of myself first, I'm happier and far less likely to react in anger or frustration. I'm more likely to give love and joy. When I feel good and have clarity, I focus on giving back to Morgan—I ask myself how I can love her better and how I should react if we bicker. I can come home and spend genuine quality time with my wife when I feel good about myself.

When I'm at work, I'm working. When it's playtime with the kids, we play; and when it's time to be with Morgan, we share our thoughts. Creating lasting change is about maintaining happiness, and a large part of that stems from the love you share with your family and, most importantly, yourself.

Do you see how the simple decision to become selfish generates happiness in your family? Do you still think everyone else needs to come first? You simply cannot live a happy life when everyone else's priorities are ahead of your own. Give yourself the gift of loving yourself first, and you will generate an abundance of happiness not only in your family life but your work life as well!

FAMILY AND TECHNOLOGY

When most people think of family time, they think it simply means everyone is at home. I want you to understand there is a difference between being at home and being *present in the moment.* Texting during dinner or scrolling through Facebook while everyone sits on the couch is *not* quality family time.

That said, I disagree with those who say we need to completely disengage from our phones or devices to engage with other people. I see YouTube, Instagram, and social media platforms as vehicles for sharing, but it's the responsibility of the family leaders to direct that activity. For example, taking phones away from your children during family time will create resentment, because they view their phones as an extension of themselves. I realize if you're over the age of thirty-five, that may be hard for you to understand.

Instead of taking phones away and creating a rift, allow them to be part of what you do together as a family. "Hey, show me that YouTube video you were telling me about. I want to see what you think of it." Ask questions that stimulate conversation and growth. "Why is this cool for you? How does this motivate you? How does this inspire you?" You can use technology to create dialogue!

In our family, we use technology on a regular basis, but there is a fine line between allowing technology and spending quality time together. My daughter is already getting a higher education by watching interactive videos and programs. When she watches those, my wife and I are right there with her, stopping the videos and doing exercises. We don't let her just sit and watch *Mickey Mouse Clubhouse* for five hours—she won't learn anything that way.

Whether we like it or not, our children are growing up in an age when technology and cell phones are the norm, and we have to embrace the times we live in. Taking away technology as punishment is like telling them they can't use their left leg and is akin to inciting a mutiny! Incorporate technology into your family time and create dialogue, but don't sit around the house with your noses buried in devices. Use technology wisely.

HOLISTIC INTEGRATION

My challenge to you is to put yourself at the top of your priority list. Yourself, your family, your friends, and your work constitute 100 percent of your happiness, and none of them work without loving yourself first.

My wife and I work fifteen to eighteen hours every day. We haven't taken a lengthy vacation together in years, but it's because we enjoy our work—we actually feel better at work than we do while on vacation! We both tend to get antsy and anxious when we're away, and we've found it's counterproductive for the growth of our relationship to put a hard line between our personal and business lives. If you love what you do and you're truly happy with your contribution to the world, it's part of who you are, and it never feels like work.

I'm not suggesting that working long days and skipping vacations will make you happy. I'm suggesting the holistic integration of your life with *you* at the core. Erase the lines between your health, business, family, and friends, while eliminating everything that doesn't help these areas evolve. If you're unhappy at work, then quit your bullshit job and follow your passion. Whose permission are you waiting for? When did you define yourself as someone who doesn't take risks? Is it your standard to remain unhappy? Haven't you always figured out solutions to your problems in the past? What makes this any different?

We get one life to live, and it does your body, mind, and spirit no good to put everyone else ahead of yourself. In order to call yourself brave, you need to practice courage. It's your own choice whether or not you are happy. Everything in your life starts and stops with you.

We are living in the greatest time in human history. Be practical! There is now more money transacted on the internet than there is in hard cash. If you can't quit your job because it pays the bills, then start a side hustle in the evenings. Put your happiness first, not your boss's.

Don't complain about not loving your career and then watch three hours of Netflix every night. You are the controller of your own destiny, and you create happiness when you have your priorities straight. I know this is a fitness book, but fitness alone will never equal happiness. Holistic integration is the only way to truly be free.

QUESTIONS FOR QUALITY TIME

When you try to *balance* work and family rather than *integrate* the two, it can feel artificial. It creates an inauthentic way of communicating, because you want to talk about the cool stuff that happened that day and the challenges you faced. This doesn't mean I sit and talk with my wife about all the problems I had that day and have a conversation that doesn't foster a connection. I talk to her about the lessons I learned, ask what she learned, and talk about how we can be stronger as a couple through what we've shared.

Morgan and I also use technology to our advantage instead of seeing it as the enemy. We've found that thirty minutes together with intelligent use of technology is better for us than sitting and watching a two-hour movie. We ask about each other's day and share pictures. We talk about what the kids did and how we can contribute more as parents, and then we Google solutions. Being engaged for thirty minutes feels far more authentic than several hours of not being present.

I urge you to embrace the times and connect through technology. Put together a specific list of questions and run through them every day to help create dialogue with your spouse, partner, or family. Spend thirty minutes asking these three questions and leverage technology to get answers.

1. How do you feel about today?
2. What can I do for you to make you feel better about today?
3. What can we do to make tomorrow better than today?

If you can answer these questions, what is naturally important to you will come to fruition. These questions are geared toward spouse/friend relationships, but they work very well with children, too.

As your children grow and your spousal relationship evolves, focus on increasing the quality of your time rather than quantity, and embrace that technology can be incorporated into that time. Since our family has started practicing these rituals, we've been able to connect and reflect on a daily basis.

As you can see, my philosophy of transforming your fitness by mastering your psychology far transcends physical activity. Happiness is the end game. A maximized quality of life doesn't happen in the weight room. Fitness is a spiritual, mental, emotional, and physical event. When you put yourself first and holistically integrate your life, you will never have to "balance" your happiness again!

★ CHAPTER 5 ★

WHEN WOULD "NOW" BE A GOOD TIME?

Time is our most precious asset, and it passes every single day. Once time is gone, we can never get it back. You'll never be able to relive this moment, be this age, or experience this season of life again. So, when is the best time to start designing your life? It's vitally important to realize how time can serve *you*, rather than you serving it.

"When would 'now' be a good time?" is a way of saying the best time to take action was yesterday. Each day that you allow life to happen *to* you is another day that you're not moving closer to the life you deserve. When will you start to eliminate everything that doesn't help you evolve? If you want to be one day closer to freedom, then don't allow the day to pass without progress. With many of my clients, fear of failure is the strongest restraint to taking action right now. This fear comes in many forms: fear of failing, fear of failing others, and fear that success will create a loss of love. Are any of these fears familiar to you?

THE *ONLY* THING YOU SHOULD FEAR IN THIS LIFE IS REGRET. AND YOU MUST BE DEATHLY AFRAID OF IT.

I'm an extremely curious person. I want to learn everything I can. Talking to people who've lived to be eighty years old and beyond will reinforce that you should fear nothing, except for failure to take risks. I've talked with many elderly people—my grandparents, my wife's grandparents, and mentors—and when I asked them for one piece of advice, they all said the same thing in different words. "Take chances, don't fear anything, and have no regrets."

When you ask them the right questions, you can compress decades of their lives into a few hours or even minutes of learning. They unanimously tell me to look out for regret, because it weighs heavy on the heart. The good news is that it's never too late.

It's okay to be fearful. Fear is a naturally occurring emotion. The beautiful thing about fear, or any emotion, is you have the power to decide what it means. The meaning we place on our emotions dictates our experience of life. Jumping out of an airplane may be scary to you, but does that fear mean you're a coward, or that you have an opportunity to be courageous? Fear is a powerful motivator, and what it means to you is 100 percent your decision. We'll always experience negative emotions, so training our brains to place an uplifting meaning on the inevitable negative ones can turn our fear into a mechanism for growth.

I'm presenting you with an opportunity to create lasting change. I'm asking you to open your mind and begin to question *why* you think the way you do. It's important to have that willingness and to truly understand the 90/10 rule: lasting change is 90 percent psychology, 10 percent execution. To create a shift in your life and enter a constant, never-ending cycle of improvement, you must believe in the 90/10 rule—this approach will give you the opportunity to ask the right questions about your current thought process. One thing I've learned through my interactions with clients and business partners is those who ask better questions will get better answers. "Should I wait until Monday to start?" is a poor question. A better one to ask ourselves is, "Why not start right now?"

ROCKING-CHAIR TEST

Imagine you're eighty years old, creaking back and forth in

an old rocker, soaking in the summer sun, and staring out over your evergreen backyard. Your great-grandchildren, who are just coming into adulthood, have the utmost respect for you. They've gathered around to listen to stories about your life and absorb lessons learned. One of them asks, "What do you regret in your life?" It's important to consider how you're going to answer this question while you still have the time to dictate the answer.

I use this process as a risk-management system for my life. When I come to a crossroads or place of uncertainty, or grow indecisive about taking action, I ask myself a simple question: would I regret not having done this if I were eighty years old? I suggest that you use this same question to determine whether or not you should take action.

Remember, life is not as complex as humans make it out to be. Practical simplicity is the key to geometric psychological growth. You don't have to understand neuroscience to design your life. I want to give you strategies that draw from science but are practical and easy to put into action.

Since you aren't in a rocking chair yet, you can still decide if you will be a role model or an example of regret. It's your choice. When looking back on your life, you'll realize that your destiny was shaped by the culmination of small decisions you made in every moment. Every choice mattered, and you were in complete control of how you spent your time.

LIFE IS LONG

After working with 20,000 different personalities, you can imagine how significantly different my case studies are. I've heard pretty much every excuse as to why fitness can't be a priority. My favorite reason for not executing healthy rituals is, "Life is short. I'm not going to eat healthily because I want to live it up while I'm here." Have you ever heard someone say this? Have you ever said this yourself?

Is life really short? In context of taking chances, risking it all, and not having any regrets, it most definitely is. Take that job promotion, start that business, marry that person, and shoot for the stars!

In the context of health, is life *really* short? How old are you? Let's say you're forty years old. Do you realize that you have a solid five decades left? With modern medicine and genetic research, you very well could have even a couple more decades than that. You're not even halfway through life yet! If you adopt the "life is short" philosophy as an excuse to live for the weekends, your life will most likely be cut short from poor moment-to-moment decisions—they'll culminate in sickness or even death. Do you want to live the next five decades with no energy or vitality? Do you want to walk around overweight and sloppy forever? You're blatantly disrespecting yourself if you're overweight, and people who tell you it's "okay" to be fat just want you to feel miserable so that they can feel better about themselves. It's not okay. It's dangerous.

I'm not suggesting it's your fault if you're part of the 70 percent of our population that's overweight, but it most certainly *is* your fault if you don't change your situation now. Your body is a gift from your creator, and it's time to start treating it like it's the greatest gift you've ever received!

The idea that life is short is clichéd bullshit. Life is long. Most people overestimate what they can do in a month and underestimate what they're capable of doing in ten years. Don't you want to see your kids, their kids, and their kids grow up? Don't you want to experience a life of fulfillment, health, and prosperity? Don't you want to feel strong, in control, and happy with your self-image?

Your body, mind, and spirit are the *only* real property you own. You have zero control over the security of your business, as the government could implement legislation that immediately takes it away. You have zero control over your house, as a tornado could rip your roof off tomorrow. What you *do* have complete control over is the meaning you associate with the events that happen in your life. The food you put into your body, the decision to be physically active, your spiritual connection, and your psychological developments are 100 percent in your control.

Life is long, and you must perceive it as such. Use your Perfect Day as a guideline for conducting yourself. You will age, and your body will change. I'm certain of that. Your body can be a pristine 1957 Chevy Bel Air convertible or a broken down, rusty one. The only difference between the latter and a smooth-running engine, glossy paint, and clean interior is the daily level of care and attention the owner puts into it. Which version of the Chevy Bel Air do you want to be in forty years?

THE 1957 CHEVY BEL AIR

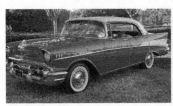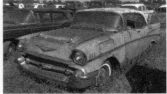

WHENEVER YOU'RE READY

Right now, I want you to find a mirror, look at your reflection, and introduce yourself to your competition. You are in complete control of *you*. Success starts and stops with *your psychology*. When you place expectations for your personal health on yourself instead of on workout programs, fad diets, or other people, you win, because it's human nature to meet our own standards. Placing your expectations on other people or events will lead to disappointment when they don't live up to them. It also gives you the opportunity to place blame. Success lies in taking ownership of your actions—there's no one to blame but yourself, because you own every decision you make. A large part of the obesity problem is that people shift blame—they don't own their decisions. It's not your kids' fault if you don't prioritize yourself first. It's not your boss's fault if you don't make time to exercise. It's not your spouse's fault for bringing processed food into the house. It's not your coworkers' fault for inviting you to lunch. It's *your* fault for allowing external circumstances to control your actions. It's *your* fault for letting your environment dictate your self-fulfillment.

It's time to stop placing blame for failure or lack of progress on external factors—these goals are yours and yours alone. It's time to take ownership of yourself.

I'm going to speak some hard truths to you, but it's only because I genuinely care. I want to see you make a life-changing decision to take ownership of all your desired outcomes. I genuinely want to help you become the best, happiest, healthiest version of yourself. I'm going to demand lot from you, because I'm certain you can do this.

Your North Star has been inside of you all along, and now that you realize its importance, you have all of the motivation you'll ever need. There are no unique or inherent talents in my clients who have achieved massive success. They've simply bought into my philosophy and taken massive action. The philosophy is so simple that it cannot be misinterpreted.

THE PHILOSOPHY MADE SIMPLE

By identifying your North Star and projecting the future pain of not reaching it, you have created an opening to transform. Then, when you fill that gap with the visualization of a Perfect Day, you've got a psychological recipe for complete lifestyle transformation.

Not *all* of my 20,000 clients have been successful, because some of them just weren't ready. Some thought I was talking crazy, some had "poor" or "good" standards, and some hadn't experienced enough pain in their lives to change. Every decision to create lasting change stems from a pain that is intolerable. That's why the best strategy to changing *right now* is to create pain and project it into the future. My commitment to my clients, and to you, is that when you are ready for change, I'm ready to guide you. But remember, the clock is ticking!

TRADE EXPECTATIONS FOR APPRECIATION

Remember, goal attainment is a process. There will be moments of joy and success, and there will also be many failures along the journey. Some days you'll feel inspired and motivated, and other days you'll feel disheartened and demotivated. There will be a healthy balance of encouragement and adversity in your journey. You've established the big goals in your life with your Perfect Day and committed to spending every waking moment attacking these goals. Now, it's time to enjoy the process of seeing things through.

You have a giant expectation of yourself, and you've done the work mentally and emotionally, so it feels like you should be there physically. The brain cannot tell the difference between vivid imagination and reality (this is called the reticular activating system—there's more to come about this later), so we tend to get impatient. The reason you must spend so much time on your Perfect Day now is because moving forward, you mustn't spend more than 5 percent of your mental energy on it. Focusing on it all day will cause impatience and unhappiness.

Remember, life is very long, and enjoying the process of goal attainment is the only way to continuously be in a beautiful state of mind. Find joy in the workouts, in the preparation of healthy food, and in the small victories along the way.

Through every step, I will remind you of the importance of enjoying the process—it creates the mentality that allows you to build on your success. There is no final destination or stopping point in your fitness journey. Daily progression equals happiness, and happiness is what we are truly after. Appreciate yourself, all that you have, and every bit of progress you make en route to attainment.

You won't care what obstacles you encounter, because you have your North Star. You know what you want and *why* you want it, and that compelling combination is a superior opponent to any hurdle in your path. What used to stop you is no match for the certainty created inside you. You have to develop an insatiable desire to reach your goals with a purpose so powerful that you can break through any limitation. Once you've made the shifts I've taught you thus far, you've won the game.

IS YOUR REALITY YOUR ACTUALITY?

It can be difficult to break free of an "it is what it is" mindset. You've been unconsciously conditioned your whole life to believe that your reality is your actuality. Your reality is what you *perceive* to be true about your life, and your actuality is what is *factually* true about it. In other words, your reality can lead you down a path of limiting beliefs, and you may never discover what could be actuality in your life. It's time to deploy the most underrated human skill—self-awareness—and learn which perspectives are perceived, as opposed to real, in your life.

We are going to erase your perception of reality and introduce you to actuality. We are going to build the self-awareness to say, "This might be my reality today, but it's not my actuality tomorrow." There's a *huge* difference between the two. The reality in our heads might be that we are overweight, we're not fitness people, we are sugar addicts, or we have no ability or skills to change our situation, because "it is what it is."

Think about those statements for a minute, and question whether they are your reality or actuality. Are they facts, or just your perception? Somewhere in the timeline of your past, you decided, "This is who I am," and it became your identity. What standard did you choose for yourself in Chapter One? If you haven't put this book down yet, you've most likely chosen to be "outstanding." The difference between great and outstanding success is a two-millimeter adjustment—in this case, becoming more self-aware.

Outstanding people make the most important adjustment every single day. They give themselves the gift of redefinition and constantly ask the question, "Is this just what I think, or is this *actually* how it is?" You're not locked into being a certain way for the rest of your life, as your identity can change with a single decision. As soon as you install this belief system, you've given yourself the opportunity to transform your fitness!

Ask yourself, "Are there other people around me in similar situations who have made the change I desire to make?" The answer is always yes. Then ask yourself, "Are they so uniquely talented, magical, and intelligent that I couldn't do the same thing?"

In the context of holistic lifestyle transformation, there is no such thing as talent. Change is never a matter of ability; it's always a matter of motivation. It doesn't matter who you are or the situation you're in—even if you have ten children and a demanding career, you can achieve life on your terms if you're self-aware and differentiate your preconditioned reality from your actuality.

Most people don't view self-awareness as an avenue to change their lives, but self-awareness holds tremendous power! Stepping outside yourself and analyzing the differences between reality and actuality allows you to see that anything is possible. However, this only works if you're willing to *tell yourself the truth!*

RUNNING TO ACTUALITY

In the early 1950s, Roger Bannister reinvented the running

world. He was a competitive middle-distance runner from Great Britain who integrated innovative training techniques that transformed the sport. He is the first major example in athletics to demonstrate the power of visualization. His goal was to be the first individual to break the four-minute mile barrier, which no human being had ever achieved. He was said to have visualized breaking this barrier night and day. Replaying the moment in his mind, he broke the four-minute mile repeatedly until it was done inside his heart and head.

Thousands of runners had tried before him, to no avail. To push himself to a higher level, Bannister ran with equally proficient pace runners. His coach taught him new strategies and made refinements to his running style so that he would be more aerodynamic and could decrease the friction between his feet and the ground. He took these physical strategies and first implemented them visually. Bannister *believed* he could do it and approached the record-breaking run with an unyielding certainty.

The reality at the time was that a sub-four-minute mile simply was not possible, and no one believed he could do it. On a foggy morning in May of 1954, Bannister would change the world forever. He took off with two pace runners, holding a blistering pace until the last 200 meters. At that point, Bannister unleashed a sprint to finish the mile in 3:59. When he broke the barrier, the previous reality of impossibility was shattered. People could no longer say a sub-four-minute mile wasn't realistic. Since the historic event, thousands of runners—from high school athletes to Olympians—have run the mile in under four minutes.

The moral of the story is what you believe to be reality isn't always actuality. If Bannister believed what everyone else had told him, he wouldn't have revolutionized mental training and created a pathway for future runners.

Most likely, somewhere out there, someone has made the same or similar accomplishment you wish to make. You might feel like you can't do it today, but that's only because you haven't done it before. It's *never* the case that you *can't* do something but rather that you just *haven't done it yet*. It's time to divorce the reality that has gotten you to a place of discontent. Are you ready to embrace the actuality of life and realize that anything is possible with enough belief? As soon as you make this distinction, your life can instantly change, because you know there's adequate potential. When you believe that change is possible, you are more likely to give a maximum effort. When effort is given, results will always follow, and achieving results will reinforce the belief in your potential, which leads to even more action!

CHAPTER 6

THE PRINCIPLES OF MENTAL MASTERY

If you thought you were going to get a ninety-day workout plan, a prescriptive meal menu, and a fixed set of rules to reach your fitness goals, you can see by now that focusing on "how to" is not my style. To create lasting change, you must master principles in the four key areas of fitness. Mental, emotional, spiritual, and physical fitness work together to design your life. In this chapter, we are going to focus on your mental fitness and specific principles you can use to build on what you've learned so far.

PRINCIPLE #1: DON'T BE A DABBLER

Have you ever met a dabbler? Someone who jumps around from gym to gym, diet to diet, and never makes a real commitment to lasting change? This person says they are going to commit to transforming their body for good, only to quit at the first sign of difficulty. They are super-motivated when it's convenient but end up failing, pivoting in direction, and starting over at the first moment of demotivation. Does this sound familiar? It's extremely easy to dabble but difficult to achieve mastery of your fitness. When you choose to do what's hard, life becomes easy, and when you choose to do what's easy, life becomes hard.

Dabblers were everywhere throughout my baseball career. Guys would get excited that the season was going to start. The enthusiastic energy from buying new cleats, purchasing a new bat, and joining a new team had them expressing how they were going to "kill it" this season. The first month of the season they were still on fire. But when the team wasn't winning games as expected and they weren't playing as much as they thought they would, their energy faded.

When this adversity hit, they reverted to statements like "I can't wait for next season" or "This isn't what I thought it would be." All of a sudden, their attitude shifted, and they were no longer the enthusiastic teammate they'd been just a month ago.

I think we can all identify dabblers in the workplace: the people who skip around from job to job and never commit to an organization. In the beginning, they are fired up and passionate about the business they're in, and they show up early for work. But when the enthusiasm wears off, they don't hesitate to take a sick day if they have a faint cough.

Beware of dabbling on your fitness journey. Our world is full of people who give up when their progression slows down. You can easily identify dabblers, as their favorite word is "plateau." But is there really such a thing as a plateau?

You've learned that even people with great standards are destined for good results at best.

THOSE WITH *OUTSTANDING* STANDARDS DON'T BELIEVE IN PLATEAUS.

Regardless of your goal, there'll eventually be slowed progression. But just because you're not making progress as fast as you did before doesn't mean it has come to a screeching halt. It simply means you must find a strategy, an insight, or a distinction that refines your approach and then continue moving forward. If you think transforming your fitness is going to be easy, you need to revisit your expectations.

Let's say you have a goal of losing twenty pounds. You buy new fitness gear, join a gym, and get a personal trainer. The excitement from your newfound motivation is at an all-time high! You show up to the gym, crush your work-outs, and follow up with a protein smoothie. This goes on for thirty days, and you lose five pounds! You're already one-fourth of the way there!

The next month is a little different. The excitement over your new program has faded, and you're sick of protein shakes. Your alarm continues to go off at the same time every day, and you find yourself becoming uninterested in early morning workouts. Thirty more days pass, and you've only lost one pound. What are you going to do?

Most people who don't understand this concept will place blame and claim their body has hit a "plateau." What you do at this critical juncture determines whether or not you're a dabbler. Are you going to blame your trainer? Your job? Your kids? That you "don't have time" anymore? Or, are you going to rip through and make the two-millimeter adjustment to reach success? Dabblers are pulled by a force greater than their stories and their blame. Since progression equals happiness and they aren't seeing it, they become unhappy and quit. Dabblers don't realize that on the other side of a so-called "plateau" is mastery and lasting change.

The next time you experience slowed progression, I want you to remember your North Star. It's critical to place your North Star somewhere visible so that you can recall it often. Make the commitment right now to use your North Star the next time you face this adversity. These moments will show up in life, and how you handle them will define your character.

DABBLING VS. MASTERY

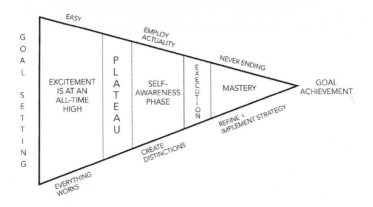

PRINCIPLE #2: REDISCOVER YOUR SUPERHERO

Remember when you were a kid, and anything was possible? Maybe you imagined being a superhero. Or maybe you wanted to be a fighter pilot, firefighter, astronaut, rock star, or fashion model. We had all sorts of audacious and outlandish ideas of who we were certain we would become. There were no limitations to those dreams, and nothing stood in the way of making them come true.

As a kid, why was it so easy to believe without borders? It's because there hadn't been time for environmental conditioning. External influences had yet to tell us we couldn't do this, or we could never be that. It might sound silly to still believe you can be a superhero, but aren't there real-life superheroes around us every day? Who is your superhero? My superheroes are my wife, Tony Robbins, Will Smith, Eminem, Gary Vaynerchuk, and Ray Dalio. They may not have laser beams shooting from their eyeballs or the ability to fly through the air, but they've certainly saved my life.

When we were young, there was nothing we could think or say that couldn't come to fruition. But somewhere along the road of growing up, somebody told us we couldn't do it. Events and judgments happened all around us, and we made a decision about who we would be based on what other people said. We let other people plant the seeds of our destiny, and we never questioned why.

I challenge you to restore your superhero mentality! How can you get back into the state of mind where you truly believe you can do anything? You had unlimited dreams and opportunities as a kid, and you still do today. Children and celebrities all have twenty-four hours each day to execute on their dreams, and the same hours are available to you as well. Whose permission do you need to take back control of your life?

Maybe you wanted to be an actor, but you didn't develop the skills early in life because someone convinced you that you weren't good at it. What's stopping you from taking acting classes today? Or your parents may have conditioned you to believe you weren't athletic, or you just "aren't an exercise person." Clients often say, "Everyone in my family is large, so it's in my genetics." This may be what they believe to be true, but it's not actuality. They certainly weren't born that way. What's stopping you from redefining yourself and questioning your preconditioning? You're a grown-ass adult, and the only person who can stop you today is yourself!

Every person on Earth is unique, and each one of us has a superpower. Statistically, you are one in 7.6 billion. You don't have to be a famous actor, NBA superstar, or Olympic athlete to achieve happiness. Everyone has the ability to be the best at something. My superpower is the ability to influence others to overcome their limiting beliefs and create lasting change in their lives.

So, what is your superpower? It lives *inside of you*. How does this relate back to your fitness goals? If you know your mind is capable of reconditioning your childhood days, then you certainly have the ability to redefine the standards for your fitness level.

I challenge you to get back into the frame of mind you had as a kid, look at your life through that lens, and give yourself the opportunity to rediscover your superpower.

You will find a refreshed sense of confidence, and you can redefine who you want to be right now. There is no law in the universe that says you can't change who you are. In fact, change is the only common denominator in life. I believe Henry Ford said it best: "Whether you think you can, or you think you can't, you're right."

PRINCIPLE #3: THE BRAIN, YOUR BRAIN, AND YOUR HEART

The brain has had one function and purpose for the last two million years: keeping the body safe. It works differently from *your* brain, and we'll distinguish between the two in a moment. The brain wants to protect us from all harm, discomfort, and pain. It doesn't take into account our level of happiness—it will do its job at all costs. The job of the heart, on the other hand, is to keep us warm, open, and fulfilled. As separate entities, the brain and heart work together, but each one doesn't understand the motivation and purpose of the other.

UNDERSTANDING HOW *"THE* BRAIN" WORKS

The brain is the first of our two brains and is shared by all human beings walking on planet Earth. Being of the same species, we share similar thoughts. We all experience worry, fear, anger, and overwhelm. People from the same generation tend to have similar problems. Our hunter-gatherer ancestors all collectively feared starvation, saber-toothed tigers, and wild bears. Skipping ahead several generations, the world collectively feared the black plague and polio. In today's world, we all collectively fear judgment, loss of love, and terrorist attacks.

It's perfectly normal for you to have thoughts like "What if I fail?" Or, "What will my friends think if I skip girls' night on Friday to go to the gym?" Or, "What if I skip lunch with coworkers and eat something healthy?" Not only are these thoughts normal, they're also inevitable. The average human on an average day will think roughly 60,000 thoughts, and studies have proven that the majority of these thoughts are negative.* However, none of these thoughts belong to you, and it's silly to allow them to control your emotions and behaviors.

UNDERSTANDING HOW "*YOUR* BRAIN" WORKS

The second brain is all yours. *Your* brain understands that *the* brain will attempt to take over your emotions. *Your* brain understands that *the* brain is physiologically designed to protect you from pain and doesn't give a shit about your happiness. *Your* brain has the ability to make conscious choices about which thoughts to hold

---

* Raj Raghunathan PhD, "How Negative Is Your 'Mental Chatter'?," *Psychology Today*, Oct. 10, 2013, https://www.psychologytoday.com/us/blog/sapient-nature/201310/how-negative-is-your-mental-chatter.

onto and which ones to let go of. *Your* brain thinks the thoughts that are specific to your life, not life in general. *Your* brain cannot do this alone—there is another part of your anatomy that is vital to ensuring that you achieve happiness: your heart.

YOUR HEART

Your heart is the bouncer at the doorway to *your* brain. Your heart decides which thoughts can join the party and which ones don't belong. Your heart is responsible for your fulfillment, happiness, and critical emotions like gratitude, joy, and appreciation. When *the* brain tells you something that doesn't align with your North Star, you must fight it with your heart! *The* brain is necessary for survival, but your commitment to the process of achieving your Perfect Day doesn't allow your "fight or flight" mentality to control your behaviors and emotions.

Right now, I want you to think of your biggest limiting belief. Give yourself a chance to be self-aware here. What thoughts are causing you to constantly fall victim to failing your fitness journey? Are these thoughts actuality or reality? Are they generated by *the* brain or *your* brain? What does your heart tell you about them? When in doubt, always follow your heart!

Visualize a giant, seven-foot Italian man standing at the

doorway of your brain, and give him a name. Let's call him Rocco. He is the bouncer to your mind who resides in your heart. Each time you notice *the* brain trying to convince you that a thought should cause negative emotions or behaviors, I want you visualize Rocco kicking the shit out of that thought! Watch him pick it up, throw it into the street, and block it so it can't get near your positivity party. Remember, you are just a bystander in this process, so enjoy the party of life!

PRINCIPLE #4: THE POWER OF FOCUS

You can take your life to a whole new level with a few simple mindset shifts. I can help you get into a peak state of mind every single day, starting right now! You have your North Star, you know what you want and why you want this transformation. We are building an army of strategies, so reaching your outcome isn't a possibility; it's a certainty. Focus is arguably the most powerful tool your brain has to offer you. Once you've mastered this principle, you are ready to conquer any challenge or obstacle on your journey to creating lasting change.

Oftentimes, we think other people are to blame when we are in unfavorable situations; we don't take ownership of our behaviors. You've already met your competition—yourself—and I'll show you how to take control of your focus in an instant. It doesn't matter if you're frustrated, overwhelmed, angry, jealous, or envious—you can use a simple thought process to shift your focus to joy, gratitude, appreciation, or delight.

THE QUALITY OF YOUR LIFE IS DETERMINED BY THE STATE OF MIND YOU LIVE IN MOST OFTEN.

It's impossible to be grateful and jealous, or angry and joyous simultaneously. Just as you learned to trade expectation for appreciation, you will learn how to trade negative emotions for positive emotions and instantly step into a positive state of mind.

How are you feeling right now? Are you open to new strategies? Maybe you are temporarily closed off. Are you in the state of mind to accept my coaching and absorb these principles? You will be able to tell how open you are if you've taken the time to *seriously* complete the North Star and Perfect Day exercises. If you haven't completed them and you're this far, stop right now, get out your pen and paper, and complete them. After all, this is your life, time, and energy you're spending with me to create lasting change. You owe it to yourself to play it all out.

I've coached people all over the world, and the reality is 80 percent of those who read this book won't take action. The 20 percent who do will change their lives forever. You don't want to be a dabbler, do you? Let's continue and fix your focus! Remember: to achieve something you've never achieved before, you have to be willing to do things you've never done before!

THE COLOR GAME

Whatever you are looking for, you will find. "Seek and you shall find," right? If you are searching for excuses, negativity, and reasons why you *can't*, you will most definitely find them. The opposite is also true. When you look for self-awareness, positivity, and reasons why you *can*, you will attract those things into your life.

To illustrate this point, I will use a demonstration. It's important that you follow along and play this fun game with me. After playing, you will understand that "whatever you focus on you will find" is a true statement.

I'd like you to look around the room, and for twenty seconds, focus as hard as you can on objects that are red. Stop reading right now and look for everything that is red. Anything that is red will count. Go!

Okay, twenty seconds is up! Now, close your eyes, and without opening them say aloud everything you saw that was red. Come on, play along! You can't change if you aren't willing to try new strategies. Do this for yourself now!

Now, with your eyes closed, name everything you saw that was the color green.

How many things could you think of that were green? If you didn't cheat, chances are you could name many more red objects than green ones. Why is that? Because I asked you to focus on red, so you found more red. Whatever you focus on you will find!

Now, once again think of all the red objects you found. Were they all really red? Or did you find some maroon objects and call them "red" to feel successful? Sometimes we fabricate what we find just so we can be right.

Since your focus was on red, your conscious choices went in that direction. If this exercise represents real life, imagine red as the stories you've told yourself as to why fitness hasn't clicked for you. If you're looking for things to blame, you will find them. You will even find maroon and call it "red," just like you will find excuses that aren't real. This is how we fall into the reality trap and become blind to actuality. What we *see* must be true, so we never question it.

Pretty deep, huh?

Your mind only has the ability to acutely focus on a few things at once. There are millions of stimuli you can focus on, but our brain isn't built that way. You would go crazy if you noticed everything, all the time. Our brains are designed to have tunnel focus. Use this power to focus on the green—in real life, the ownership of your fitness goals. You'll rarely find negativity if you search for positivity. This simple game shows that when you look for reasons to succeed or fail, you will inevitably find them. *You completely own* the choice of what to look for.

RETICULAR ACTIVATING SYSTEM (RAS)

Our brains are equipped with an amazing tool called the reticular activating system (RAS). This small part of your brain is a network of neurons located in the brain stem. Practically speaking, it allows whatever we visualize to become our reality. This vital part of our mind enables us to focus on what is important to us. Whatever you think about during the day you will most definitely find. When fitness success is important to you, you'll find ways to make it happen. When fitness success isn't important, you'll find the excuses to justify why you're not doing it.

The RAS can be an extraordinary tool if you understand how to use it. On the other hand, it can take your fitness journey into a downward spiral if used inappropriately. Have you ever noticed how a pessimist is rarely disappointed in not reaching their goals? They let their RAS block everything out of their life that could be good, and they fail to realize how much better life could be. They have a world of possibilities in front of them, but they can't find what they aren't looking for.

Have you ever bought a brand-new pair of shoes that you really dug? Or a brand-new car that you fell in love with? What happens during the subsequent days after purchase? You begin to notice everyone who has the exact same item you have. You thought your Chevy Tahoe was the only one in town; then, you pulled out of the lot and passed five of them on your way home. The car (or shoes) became important to you, so you started to notice them, even though they were there all along.

In fact, your RAS is responsible for you picking up this book and reading it. Your health is extremely important to you, so you sought ways to become a healthier person, whether consciously or unconsciously.

For example, asking, "How did I get to this bad place in my life?" is a negative question, with a negative focus. When you ask questions like this, you will find the answers and notice all the reasons why you are in a bad place. This is the source of the excuses and false stories of your reality. It does no good to focus your energy on problems from a negative perspective.

You must ask yourself the better question, "How am I going to take control of my life?" Ask positive questions, and you'll get positive answers. This is precisely where resolve comes from. Allowing your RAS to attract what's important will solve the issue rather than compound reasons to feel bad about yourself.

If your focus is on "why me," you'll point blame at your family, upbringing, or other circumstances in your life. But if your focus is on "why not me," that additional word in the middle eliminates every possible excuse—you'll realize you don't need anyone's permission to pursue your fitness journey with full confidence.

Your mind is very powerful. What you focus on most of the time is what you will become. It's your decision where to place your focus, and every decision moves you closer to or further away from your destiny—your Perfect Day.

PRINCIPLE #5: THE FIVE-MINUTE RULE

I have a principle that offers a little grace as we go through this journey together. It's called "the five-minute rule." Can I be straightforward with you for a moment? Even with a clearly defined North Star, your Perfect Day ingrained into your central nervous system, and the power of focus on your side, you will slip up, fail, and face adversity. But I have some exciting news for you: it's perfectly fine! Isn't that a relief? You must expect failure, and when you encounter it, you have to realize it's merely opportunity in disguise.

There's no such thing as perfection. In fact, perfectionists are the unhappiest people in the world. Earlier, I mentioned the only fear you should have is regret, but if I had to choose a second one, it would be perfectionism. Striving for perfection leads to your ultimate failure. I'm going to introduce the five-minute rule, which is a tool you will use when you encounter failure. You'll learn from it and move forward without beating yourself up.

The name of this principle sounds similar to the time-honored "five-second rule" you follow when you drop food on the floor. If you pick it up in time, it's still okay to eat it! However, my five-minute rule is much different. With this principle, you give yourself five minutes to feel overwhelmed, frustrated, or sorry for yourself, and after those five minutes have passed, you snap back to living your life with purpose. You can be angry or sad for five minutes, but that's it!

You can 100 percent count on facing uphill battles throughout your journey. Failures are inevitable, but they are your most powerful weapon. Failure doesn't shape your character, but the way you handle failure does. Nobody likes to expect failure, but all of my successful fitness clients understand that short-term failures are necessary to reach the long-term manifestation of their goals. There are no mistakes in life, only lessons.

I used to have a bad habit of dwelling on past mistakes. I'd overplay scenarios in my mind, go down rabbit holes, and constantly mull over "what ifs." I manifested them into much bigger issues—I'd compare the phenomenon to hallucinating. Have you ever done this? If you have, you know it's a continuous cycle, and it can lead to paranoia or general surliness.

In my parking lot days, an internet troll wrote a nasty review about Morgan and me for buying a Range Rover. They said we were "money hungry and didn't care about our clients." Furthermore, they wrote that Morgan was a "bitch," and I was a "dumb meathead who favors good-looking women in the gym."

Anyone who actually knew us understood that these claims were far from the truth, and they could clearly see this troll was unhappy with their own life. But we were twenty-four years old when this happened, and our emotional maturity was nowhere near what it is today. We thought that since this person wrote bad things about us, everyone would believe them. We started making shit up in our heads and going over all of the "what ifs," and it caused some serious pain. We commented back to the troll, and it fueled the fire of the negative thread. Maybe we never should have posted a picture of our new ride on Instagram, but the real failure was allowing people we didn't even know to affect us psychologically.

This experience taught me an important lesson. I vowed to never again spend that much mental energy on someone who didn't know me at all. Morgan and I decided that our belief in what we wanted to accomplish was so strong that a thousand internet trolls couldn't dent the shield of belief we had in ourselves. If someone who actually knew me said those things, I would pay attention. Otherwise, I would let strangers sip their "haterade," and I'd keep moving forward.

I used this error in judgment as an opportunity to incorporate the five-minute rule into my life. Today, if I make a mistake, whether big or small, I give myself five minutes to complain, dwell, or be frustrated. From there, I visualize my seven-foot-tall Italian mind-bouncer beating my negative thoughts into the ground and kicking them to the curb. Then, I move forward. I don't dwell on the past, and I don't waste valuable mental space feeling bad about myself, especially if it's because someone else is unhappy with their own life. Misery loves company, and the crabs in the bucket will always attempt to pull you back in.

I encourage you to adopt this tactic on your fitness journey. Whether you're a business leader orchestrating key moves in a company or a rock star mom at home, you can apply this principle to your life. A mother is often a household's CEO, and there are days when her baby's crying, her toddler is coloring on the wall, the dog is pooping on the carpet, her twelve-year-old daughter is talking back, and everyone in the house is "hangry." It's chaos in full stride! What approach should this mom take? Throw up her hands and give up? Crumble under the stress? Yell at the kids, or smack them in the butt? Resent them for their behavior?

This mom has a choice to make. She can let the kids' behavior ruin her day, or she can realize that babies are supposed to cry, her walls will eventually experience all colors of the rainbow, and twelve-year-old girls are—well, they're challenging, and dogs poop on floors. It means her family is normal, and she can take five minutes to feel frustrated. Then, she must trade the expectations she has of her family for appreciation of this season of life.

PRINCIPLE #6: YOUR BIOGRAPHY IS NOT YOUR DESTINY

Looking back at your past, do you see situations where you could have applied the first few principles of this book? Now that you have these tools and distinctions, do you see how you could have used them five, ten, or twenty years ago? It's great if you can see it, but that's not why

I asked this question—I want you to consider the *impact* of these tools.

Whether your past is dark like mine, it's darker than mine, or you had a wonderful upbringing, you picked up this book for a reason, and you've invited me to be your coach. I don't want you to erase your past, but I do want to question any false standards or preconditioning that your past, parents, siblings, or job set for you. Your past is part of who you are, but it doesn't determine who you're going to be!

I will continue to reinforce the fact that my teachings will transcend fitness. Fitness is the perfect metaphor for every area of your life. The mental principles that I'm teaching can be applied to parenting, entrepreneurship, financial freedom, and your spiritual relationships—any realm of life.

THE ELEPHANT IN THE ROOM

Are you familiar with how a circus elephant is trained? When a baby elephant is small and weak, she's tied to a rope attached to a wooden stake. She tries to rip free, but the rope is too strong. Eventually, she's convinced she's not strong enough to break free, and she stops trying.

Years later, when the elephant is strong and weighs six tons, she is still easily constrained by a light rope and wooden stake, because her past has conditioned her to think it's impossible to break free. The elephant learns this limitation when she's small and weak, and this lesson follows her into adulthood. She is convinced that what was once true will *always* be true. She remains imprisoned by her limiting beliefs, when clearly, she has the strength to pull the stake out of the ground and free herself.

Isn't that interesting? The truth is that some of us are just like big powerful elephants who have been conditioned by our pasts to be weak and powerless. In what areas of your life are you convinced you can't break free? It's never true that you can't. You possess the absolute and infinite power of the universe, and you can do whatever you believe you can do.

To break free, you must first realize that a belief is nothing more than a thought you keep thinking. How do you change a disheartening thought into an empowering one? You can easily transform your beliefs by choosing different thoughts. Rocco the mind-bouncer really comes in handy here. The only limitations on your life experience are the boundaries of your beliefs.

If you've bought into lack and limitation, you will suffer. If you believe that "it is what it is," you'll be imprisoned by your societal, parental, or spousal conditioning. Repetition of thoughts leads to belief, and belief leads to physical manifestation. If you've been taught to be less than you're truly worth, a new set of empowering beliefs is all you need to be set free!

The fix is simple.

ANYTIME YOU HEAR YOURSELF USING THE WORDS "I CAN'T," TRADE THEM OUT FOR "I HAVEN'T YET," AND YOU WILL CHANGE YOUR THOUGHTS.

Change your thoughts, and change your beliefs. Change your beliefs, and change your life.

Turn "I can't seem to lose the weight" into "I haven't been able to lose the weight *yet*." Stating this thought from a presumptive position begins to condition your mind that you can; you simply haven't figured it out yet.

When you change your language, you make a promise to yourself to think thoughts in a positive and presumptive manner. When positive affirmations are repeated, they will become your reality and what you know to be true. When you're certain that you can, you'll reclaim your freedom, and you'll be able to conquer anything you desire. Your actuality is that you can escape the prison of limiting beliefs, and it's your choice whether or not you do so. You're not a trapped elephant, and if you've been acting like one, it's time to rip that stake out of the ground and run free.

YOU WEREN'T BORN THIS WAY

We all have a story. Where we came from, how we were raised, family life, and friends are important parts of our stories. Whether it was sunshine and roses or struggle and strife, our past does not dictate our future. Many of us have allowed other people to determine a standard for our life that is far too low. My goal is for this book to become your saving grace and to inspire you to adopt these principles, move to action in your own life, become a master, and then teach others.

The truth is, no one is born overweight. No one is born a sugar addict. No one is born bad or lazy. No one is born with the inability to transform their psychology and master their fitness. Your limiting beliefs were developed through your upbringing and are now maintained by the people you choose to surround yourself with. Give *yourself* the permission to decide what's next. Don't wait for anyone else to grant you access to a maximized quality of life. Doesn't this shit fire you up? By now, there should be a giant boulder lifted from your shoulders. Now, it's time to squat press this thing and achieve some fitness goals!

There's no end to the stories about people who came from

nothing and became wildly successful entrepreneurs. Oprah Winfrey is a perfect example. She endured physical and sexual abuse as a child and then became pregnant as a young teenager. She never had the baby because she miscarried. Can you imagine the emotional stress placed on a young girl enduring such life conditions? Every card in the deck was stacked against her, and it appeared she was destined to become a product of her horrible environment.

However, Oprah did just the opposite. She single-handedly disrupted the television industry, redefined success, and became the first female African American billionaire. She overcame her circumstances and climbed from one side of the socioeconomic scale to the other, despite a society that favored white males. Her story provides inspiration to many and shows anything is possible.

How did Oprah do it? Did she have some magical skill that helped her beat the odds? No, she didn't. Obviously, she's talented, and that led her to a prominent place in front of the camera, but it was her *psychology* that led to her success. Your superpower may not be the same as Oprah's, but you *do* have one. Everyone has a skill, a superpower, or a "secret sauce" that no one else has. If you believe that, you can leverage that power, set a new standard, and be successful in your fitness—and whatever else you choose!

I grew up in a low-income neighborhood in Battle Creek,

Michigan. My parents were physically and verbally abusive to each other and to their children. To this day, I see images of my father punching my mother and her punching right back. I also vividly remember my dad throwing me down the stairs and slamming my head through drywall. I don't bring this up again for your sympathy but rather to remind you I'm living proof that your biography is not your destiny.

REWRITING YOUR STORY

How would you have coped in a situation like mine or Oprah's? Would you have mustered up the courage to get up and move into another day or succumbed to your circumstances? Whatever your background, you don't have to accept it as "the way it is." You can't change your past, but you can certainly change what your past *means*. I challenge you to rewrite the first chapter of your story, because your life's book isn't published until your physical body is gone.

How do you view your life story? Is it a coloring book or a blank canvas? If you see it as a coloring book, you'll always stay within the lines, never take risks, and let the page define your art. You are free to decide which colors to use, and you might end up with a nice picture, but it's not truly yours—it was illustrated by someone else.

If you see your life as a blank canvas, it gives you the

opportunity to open up your imagination, and there are no limits to what you can create. You can light up the world with a new business, create your dream home, or be the champion of a sport—you can exceed your fitness goals on your own terms. Your imagination shines outside the lines. The only limitation you have in this life is your own imagination!

I challenge you to view your life's book with blank pages. You are the author of your own story, and the next page is limited only by your imagination. It doesn't matter how old you are or if you write the next page today, tomorrow, or next year. You'll make the change when you want it badly enough. Make the commitment at this moment to write your story the way you want it—how you want your legacy to be remembered.

Growing up, I didn't get to decide who my parents were. In fact, if I had to do it over again, I wouldn't change a thing. I've forgiven my parents for the way they've treated me and will always have love for them. I am proud to be the person I am today. If you're going to blame your parents for everything they *didn't* do, you'd better give them credit for what they *did* do. I have, and it's the only way I've been able to find peace, rewrite my story, and choose the meaning I've given my background.

Remember, life is happening *for* you—use adversity as

a tool to fuel success. Finding Tony Robbins' *Personal Power* CD was the defining moment in my life that led me to understand what I needed to do. It taught me the importance of psychology to create positive change. You must realize that your story is far from over, life is long, and you have decades left to live. It's never too late, you're never too old, and you're never too far gone to generate a life of health and happiness that you and your family can be proud of.

You get one life. You get one opportunity to be great.

WE MUST ALL SHOOT FOR THE STARS. WE DON'T ALWAYS REACH OUR GOALS, BUT IF WE FALL SHORT, WE STILL LAND ON THE CLOUDS.

Your journey to fitness isn't about slaying your goals; it's about understanding that ultimate health and happiness are in your complete control. One life is all we need when we live it to the fullest.

DO YOU. BE DIFFERENT. BE AUTHENTIC.

Society conditions most of us to think we should go to college, get a degree, get a job, get married, buy a house, have kids, and have a traditional family/work life. The follow-the-crowd plan is for people who are unwilling to be bold. Life is so much more fulfilling on *your* terms. It's natural human behavior to live up to the standards you've set for yourself, so when you have outstanding standards, you will inherently do outstanding things. Don't do yourself, your family, and your creator a disservice by setting the bar too low or trying to be like someone else.

Long ago, I decided I wasn't going to be like my parents, and my future family wouldn't go through what I did. However, this decision to be different went beyond my immediate family and environment—I dedicated my life to ending pain for others and to giving families all over the world the opportunity to experience lasting change. I've been able to impact hundreds of thousands of people in many different countries through my gyms, YouTube, Instagram, Facebook, the Burn Boot Camp webpage and blog, and numerous media outlets. You can use your past as fuel for a creative fire and have an impact on the world, or you can accept and settle for the status quo—the choice is yours. If I had let my biography influence my destiny, I wouldn't be coaching you today!

SPECIFIC IMPACTFUL MOMENTS

All of this is powerful, isn't it? Do you feel like you can do anything by now? I know you're excited about digging into the process, but I made a promise of practicality I intend to keep. I would never suggest *what* you should do without suggesting *how* to do it.

LIFE CHANGING EXERCISE: REDEFINE YOUR PAST RIGHT NOW

Think of moments in your past that have been the most impactful or influential. These moments are always connected to a strong emotion, because emotion creates *motion*. For example, I want you to visualize exactly where you were, who you were with, and how you felt on 9/11 after those planes crashed into the World Trade Center. There was great emotion attached to that day. Now, tell me where you were on 10/11. You most likely don't remember, unless that was a special day for you, because there was no emotion attached to it.

Now, I want you to think of the most significant emotional moment in your past—something that created a deep sense of pain inside of you. I'm going to give you the opportunity to redefine your ability to create the lasting change you desire, if you're willing to play it all out with me.

What distinct moment in your past guided the definition of your fitness ability? Go back to that place. Don't just think about it—feel the emotions you felt when this event occurred. How did this play into your view of what you can accomplish today? Have you used this moment to create complacency because you are scared to fail? Have you not taken the leap into a fit life because it would make people you love feel bad about themselves? What is it about this event that was significant to defining your fitness?

Once you have an event in mind, it's time to give it a new meaning by answering the following questions.

★ What are you focusing on?
★ What does this focus mean?

Start by using the example of "why me" vs. "why not me." Change a subtlety about this event that allows you to create new meaning that aligns with your North Star. You can use the sample below to further guide your thought process.

Sample Exercise

Let's say the defining event that created limiting beliefs is when your father said you were "big-boned."

★ What do I focus on?

Limiting Belief: *I'll never be fit, because it's in my DNA to be overweight.*

New Empowering Belief: *I know other overweight people who have lost more weight than I have to lose. It must be possible. This may be my past reality, but my new actuality is that I can do this.*

★ What does this focus mean?

Limiting Belief: *I shouldn't even attempt to work out and eat healthily, because I'm destined to be this way. It is what it is.*

New Empowering Belief: *Since losing weight is possible, I will use this belief to begin my journey today. It will have ups and downs, but I'm certain I can do it. It's already done inside of me, and it will take consistency and perseverance to see it physically.*

Use this sample as a guide to create new empowering beliefs about your fitness. Reading through this one time might not suffice. You cannot create motion in your life without tapping into your emotions, so I suggest you stop here and read through the sample exercise over and over, until you create emotion inside your body. Doing this is vitally important to creating emotion inside of your body. Visualize how this past event made you feel over and over again, and then take the time to associate a new empowering meaning to it.

Please, take this seriously, as it could change the course of your life forever. Repeat the new meaning aloud twenty times a day for thirty days, with conviction in your voice to lock it in. Do this, and you'll never be the same again!

★ CHAPTER 7 ★

THE PRINCIPLES OF EMOTIONAL MASTERY

Mental and emotional principles are closely related. Now that you have all the skills, knowledge, and beliefs to master your mentality, we will shift our focus to emotional mastery. Mental mastery is your ability to control the way you think and ultimately control your outcomes. Emotional mastery focuses on how positive or negative thoughts make you feel. Emotional mastery is your ability to control your *feelings*.

Do you realize that we have yet to talk about strategies for working out, eating right, and mastering your physical appearance? I would be doing you a disservice to introduce you to diet plans and exercises right off the bat. After all, haven't you tried starting with the "how to" many times before, only to fail?

My mission is to help you stop starting over, and emotional mastery is a vitally important part of this process. Successful people do what unsuccessful people aren't willing to do, even when they don't *feel* like doing it. This section is going to teach you how to stop negotiating with your brain and train you to do what you say you're going to do, when you say you're going to do it.

PRINCIPLE #1: YOUR DAILY PREGAME

I'm an athlete, but my playing days are over, so I view my personal health and my businesses as my sporting events, and every day is practice. You would never play a game without warming up, would you? So why should we treat life any differently?

Generally speaking, what do most of us do before we go to bed? We stare at that box on the wall, watching other people live their lives or tuning in to the latest world crisis. Then, when we get up in the morning, what's the first thing we usually do? Before we even get out of bed, we roll over, grab our phone, read news stories, check our email, or read text messages. We start our day focused on yesterday's problems or today's bad news. No wonder the world is such a negative place! The people living in it are exposed to negativity at the beginning and end of each day. We need a strategy to filter this exposure, and if we sit around waiting for the world to show us good, we'll be waiting a lifetime.

We're adults, and we have the power to decide what we expose ourselves to. You're on the fast track to a bad day if you don't know how to filter your exposure. Are you going to be motivated for your workout that morning if you roll over and immediately start putting fires out at work? If your focus immediately shifts to the problems in your life, how do you think you'll perform that day? Where does your focus go when this happens?

The unfortunate truth is that most of us default to these behavioral patterns, and it's secretly causing us anxiety, stress, and overwhelm. You need a strategy in place to have gratitude and appreciation in your life first thing in the morning—this is the only way to dictate the way you play the game of life every day.

For most of my life, I was a victim of "wake and text," which killed my positive vibe for the entire day. I scrolled through Instagram, focused on what I *didn't* have, and never stopped to appreciate what I *did* have. When I became self-aware enough to see that these patterns were affecting my quality of life, I knew something had to change.

Whether it's the morning, afternoon, or evening, your focus can be adjusted within a few short minutes. Pregaming is something that has changed my life, and I know it will change yours, too!

THE MOST IMPORTANT TIME OF YOUR LIFE

The most important time of your life is when your alarm goes off every morning.

Your entire day is predicated on what you do for the first ten or fifteen minutes after waking up. If you get up in the morning and think, "Ugh, I don't want to get up and work out," how much effort do you think you'll put toward that day's fitness goals? And even if you do get up and "sort of" work out, it's not sustainable behavior, because you don't enjoy it. If you're prying yourself out of bed every day, starting with negative thoughts and halfhearted efforts, you won't get results.

World-renowned motivational speaker and life coach Mel Robbins has a solution to get you out of bed in the morning. She has an activation energy tactic called the "5 Second Rule" (not to be mistaken for my Five-Minute Rule). Her rule sounds extremely simple, because it is, and this one minor insight can change the way you function every day. The rule is this: as soon as you open your eyes, count down from five. When your countdown reaches "one," simply get up. This sounds too good to be true, right?

The simplest strategies always work the best. Isn't getting up in the morning an important step toward your achieving your North Star? The more you repeat this, the more it will become a habit. Make a commitment to stop negotiating with yourself, and use the 5 Second Rule to catapult yourself out of bed for ten straight days—this will lock in the habit. No more negotiating with yourself!

Your North Star must be more important to you than pressing the snooze button. Revisit your standards, and remember that those with outstanding standards will create discipline. When the pain of failing to reach your goals is greater than the comfort of sleeping in, you will get up!

Choose your "hard"! It's hard being unmotivated, lazy, and out of shape. It's also hard to get up, work out, and eat right every day. Nothing in life that is worth doing is easy! Either way, life is hard, and you choose which route you take.

If you're this far into the book, you know what you want and why you want it. Your North Star should create the hunger to change your life—it should motivate you. But if you're just starting out and struggling with change, the following strategies will help eliminate repeated failure with getting your day started.

LOSE THE SNOOZE

If the temptation to hit the snooze alarm is initially too great, you need to remove that temptation. I highly suggest reading Mel's book *The 5 Second Rule*. It will provide you with tools to seize the day, use activation energy to stop negotiating with your brain, and begin following your North Star.

Not sure you have the discipline to leap out of bed in five seconds? Then let's remove that problem from the equation entirely! Move your alarm clock to the other side of the room. While you're at it, plug your phone in over there, too. This will force you to get out of bed in the morning to turn off the alarm and check your phone. It's important to take an action that signals to your brain "I don't go back to sleep after this happens." You're up, so go ahead and make the bed (or your side of it, if someone else is still sleeping). Making the bed tells your subconscious you've started the day, and it's time to get moving.

Getting up is simple, and you've won the first battle of the pregame when you do that instead of hitting snooze. Then, you can ignite your physiology through your vocal chords. Throw three fist-pumps into the air and say, "I won!" or something similarly playful. This gives your brain the signal that you're ready to meet the day, and it reinforces positive behavior so that you'll crave more.

WAKE UP TO ACTUALITY

The reality is that you'll be tired when you first get up. People often say, "I'm just so tired in the morning." Welcome to the club! This is *the* brain talking, and you must realize how silly this sounds. Everyone is tired for the first few minutes of the day, whether they've slept for six hours or fifteen.

You think you're the only one who's not a morning person? Time to wake up! Is anyone even *born* a morning person? Does anyone get up at 4:30 a.m. every day for their entire life because they just love it so much? I don't know anyone who enjoys getting up at 4:30 in the morning. I sure don't! Find me someone who physically enjoys getting out of bed before 5:00 a.m., and I'll show you a liar. What I enjoy is the feeling I get from following my heart and not allowing *the* brain to talk me into oversleeping. I enjoy the sense of pride I have from getting more work done in a single day than most people do in a week. I enjoy the confidence I get from doing what I put my mind to.

I'd rather sleep until 8:00 a.m., but sleeping another four hours doesn't align with my goals. I have to get up and work out before my kids wake up. As soon as they're up, I have to tend to them, and the day kicks into high gear. My day consists of spending time with family, training clients, running my businesses, and kicking ass! I wasn't born a morning person, but I have made the decision to die as one!

MORNING ENERGY HACK

If you tend to sleep way too long, make a caffeinated green tea drink before you go to bed. Don't drink it at night; set the cup on your nightstand. When you get up the next morning to walk across the room and shut off the alarm, drink the tea. Try going back to sleep after chugging caffeine-laced tea! Your body won't let you—it's lit up and wants to get moving!

HOW TO PREGAME LIKE THE PROS

I know we're all busy people. We're moms, dads, business leaders, teachers, students, volunteers, and doctors. Early morning might be the only time you have to yourself—it's important to take control of what you think about and reflect upon what's meaningful to you. Pregaming prepares your mind and psychology to take on the day from a beautiful, positive perspective that is self-generated, rather than from the negative perspective the world is constantly force-feeding you.

The first ten to fifteen minutes of the day are about getting your mind right for what's ahead. Every happy person I've had the chance to speak with practices a morning ritual that allows them to control their emotions. They don't let CNN's newsfeed get the best of them, look at the crashing stock market, or dive into work-related problems as soon as they wake up. That bullshit isn't going anywhere, and you can tend to it once you've taken care of your number one priority: yourself.

MY MORNING ROUTINE

When the pain of not living up to my standards weighed more than the temptation of sleeping in, waking up when my alarm went off became easy. This is why taking the opportunity to constantly reevaluate your standards and concisely identify a North Star is so important. I made a decision to completely change my rituals and have practiced them every single day since.

I moved my phone and alarm across the room, and I put a tea drink on my nightstand every night. I follow the routine we discussed above to the letter: get up, drink the tea, and make the bed. Then, I put on fitness gear and clothing, and I head out for a light twenty-minute jog. This is now my default pattern, and it has been positively reinforced through the result of these behaviors: increased productivity.

You don't always have to enjoy working out, but positively associating the feelings you get from it will keep you focused and excited about repeating the behavior. If you choose to follow this ritual, it might be easy to look out the window on a rainy day and think, "Well, I'll get soaked. I'm not going out for a jog." Or on a cold and snowy day, you may not feel like putting multiple layers on. It can always be too hot, too windy, too cold, or too wet. There's always an excuse if you want one. Whatever you focus on you will find. Unless the weather might cause me physical harm, there's nothing stopping me.

Admittedly, there are days when outside influences steer me away from my rituals, but I never forget they are a part of me—I know I'll come back to them. Even when the snow is four feet deep and will take weeks to melt, I know I'll be back. I simply modify my strategy for the time being. It's important to hold true to rituals and return to them after distractions or roadblocks inevitably come your way.

THREE PREGAME QUESTIONS

The point of this immediate wake-up call followed by a light jog is not to practice physical fitness but rather emotional fitness. There is a specific emotional ritual I practice that incorporates three questions to pregame my day. I speak the questions one at a time and focus on each one for five minutes. It's okay to ask them silently in your head, but I find when I say them aloud it works like an incantation, and I *feel* the emotions. Below are the three questions I ask myself every morning on my light run, and I encourage you to practice this ritual as well. It ties mental and emotional fitness together and has single-handedly taken my life to incredible heights.

Question One

The first question is "What am I grateful for in my life?" You might balk at this question, thinking you're in such a bad place you have nothing to be grateful for. If this is you, put that negativity aside for a moment. If nothing else, you live in a country with endless opportunities to pursue. It's emotionally impossible to be grateful and fearful at the same time. Keep digging until you have an answer—there *is* something! Maybe it's your children, spouse, career, or relationship with a higher power. When you ask yourself this question, you realize that even in times of perceived struggle or hopelessness, there is always something to be grateful for, and that will make you smile.

Really take the time to vividly imagine what you're grateful for. How does this make you feel? Think of a specific moment when you were so filled with gratitude that you got emotional. Take yourself back to this place for a moment. It can be something simple like feeling the wind on your face as you run or even the physical ability to run down the street. For five minutes, continue to feel how tremendously grateful you are.

Question Two

The second question is "Who do I love the most, and who loves me the most?" Think of one or two people you love more than anything and who will always love you in return, regardless of any personal decisions you've made or will make. Focus on how that love makes you feel, and connect to those emotions. It's emotionally impossible to feel love and anger simultaneously.

When I stop and ask myself who I love and who loves me, I envision my heart as a soft, open place that continues to expand. With every deep breath, it gets softer and wider, and it increases my capacity to love. I begin to feel emotions that are in alignment with the people I love and how it makes me feel when I smell, touch, hear, and kiss them. Life centers on love, and as you focus on it, you let more of it into your heart. This focus builds great appreciation for the special relationships you have, and you can't help but start your day off appropriately.

Question Three

The third question is "In six to twelve months, what goals will I accomplish?" This question allows space for the process of visualization. While envisioning your goals, you must see them as done and have certainty they will be accomplished. Your brain cannot tell the difference between actuality and imagination; therefore, this conditioning process manifests itself physically over time. By accomplishing your goals repeatedly in your mind, you are far more likely to reach them.

By answering these three questions and going for a twenty-minute run, you'll give yourself the chance to feel grateful, loving, appreciative, joyous, and proud, while washing away any anger, frustration, overwhelm, or discontent. I highly recommend physical movement combined with emotional stimulation, because it's a powerful way to connect with these emotions. This ritual allows you to practice physical, mental, emotional, and spiritual fitness, while simultaneously compounding feelings of fulfillment.

DOING IT YOUR WAY

Maybe you're thinking, "I like to run at night." Maybe you don't like running at all and prefer alternate forms of exercise. That's no problem, because there are multiple strategies for everything. You don't have to get up early and do what I do. It's just an example of a ritual—the one that works for me. I want you to do what's right for *you*!

If you love early mornings and choose meditation as your

first activity of the day, you can ask the three questions during your time of solitude. But if you prefer to exercise over your lunch hour and listen to a podcast because it helps you stay in a work mindset, obviously the early morning routine doesn't align with your Perfect Day. Well, surely, you're going to shower before work. Use that time to close your eyes and grab a moment of solitude under the warm water. Take advantage of feeling relaxed and fresh, and move into a state of positivity.

Maybe you don't shower in the morning; you just get up and head straight to work. You can use the commute time for solitude. Instead of listening to the radio, ask and practice visualizing the answers to the three questions. If you get up and like to lift weights, use the time between sets to breathe and focus on your pregaming.

There are several environments and times of day in which you can practice this strategy. Regardless of who you are and the goals you've established, the process gives your life perspective. It innately eliminates fear, anger, and frustration. I guarantee you'll feel amazing after answering these questions. You'll automatically trade appreciation for expectation, and your mind, body, and spirit will connect on a level you've never felt before!

RECREATE MEANING

You know that your focus goes where your attention flows. We have the power to choose what to focus on—we have control over the destiny of our lives. Furthermore, we have the power to decide what that focus *means* in our lives.

EVERY EVENT THAT OCCURS IN OUR LIVES, POSITIVE OR NEGATIVE, IS ASSOCIATED WITH THE MEANING YOU CHOOSE TO GIVE TO IT.

The event happens, and you can decide to focus on a meaning that empowers you—or one that disempowers you. In other words, the meaning you place on the event controls the way you feel, and the way you feel determines your experience of life. You have the power to *choose* the meaning you give to life's events or circumstances; therefore, you have the power to design your life experience.

Let's say you've had a failed attempt to lose weight in the past. For this example, the goal is to lose twenty pounds in three months. You joined a Burn Boot Camp gym and your motivation was at an all-time high. You executed what you thought to be a solid strategy to attain this goal. You worked out hard, consumed clean foods, and completed your one-on-one meetings with your trainer. At the end of three months, you'd only lost three pounds.

So, for this event, you set out to lose twenty pounds but

only lost three. What will you choose to focus on? You can focus on the disciplines, good habits, and consistency that helped you lose three pounds, or you can focus on the numbers that suggest you failed.

What's the experience of your health journey going to look like when you focus on what you've accomplished? You'll feel a sense of pride and progression that creates confidence. Increased confidence will give you the momentum you need to continue your journey. You never have to start over again, because you've created a positive neurological association with great rituals.

What's the experience like when you focus on what you *didn't* accomplish? You'll feel a sense of disappointment and frustration that breeds resentment toward a perfectly good strategy. You'll create a negative association with new habits and become disenchanted with the process. Time will pass, you'll once again experience pain from the way you look and feel, and you'll start over again.

The meaning you place on events will shape your view of the world. When associating events with negative meanings, you'll create a reality in your head that is inconsistent with the actuality surrounding you. Do you get it now? This is why success is 90 percent psychology and 10 percent strategy.

SUCCESS VS. FULFILLMENT

I believe there's a tremendous difference between success and fulfillment. Most people think of success and instantly envision monetary wealth. Although financial success is one element, I know many millionaires who are miserable. Money doesn't equal happiness. I define fulfillment as an abundance of gratitude, appreciation, thankfulness, love, and joy. Fulfillment is a mindset, and without it, life cannot be physically or emotionally fulfilling. Tony Robbins says, "Success without fulfillment is the ultimate failure."

Just as each person has a unique set of fingerprints, no two people have the same definition of fulfillment. You must understand the contrast between fulfillment and success, and then define what makes *you* happy. If you meet a weight-loss goal because you think you need to look like a photoshopped woman on Instagram, you won't be fulfilled—you lost the weight for the wrong reasons. You must resolve to reach your goals for the reasons that are fulfilling to you, in a way that's fulfilling to you, not to someone else. We have to stop trying to live other people's lives and start designing our own. The emotions you feel are responsible for fulfillment, and fulfillment is an art.

TRANSFORMATIVE LANGUAGE

Have you ever noticed the way you talk to yourself? Are you aware of your words, and do you realize their impact? The language you use influences and intensifies the emotions you feel. There are blatant and obvious transformational words that we use, and they create an entirely new meaning to what we say.

For example, "I'm starving right now. I could eat a cow!" Let's take a look at this through the lens of actuality. Are you really starving? Chances are you have enough body fat to feed yourself for seven days without eating. Is it really possible to eat a whole cow? Clearly it isn't. What you really mean to say is "I'm feeling a little bit hungry, and eating something might be a good idea." See the difference? The word "starving" intensifies the feeling of hunger, and using it gives your subconscious permission to chow down. We have more conversations with ourselves than any other human being, and it's very important to deploy self-awareness and be extremely careful what we say to ourselves.

There are also more subtle ways in which we use transformative language patterns. This type of language can ruin the opportunity to create lasting change. Our example of "I can't" vs. "I haven't yet" is a great one. Using words like *if*, *try*, or *hope* automatically creates doubt and uncertainty. "I hope I can lose the weight" is an example you may hear often. By eliminating a single word, "hope," you change the entire meaning of what you said. Hope is a bad strategy for reaching your fitness goals. Life is black and white; either you do, or you don't.

Frequent use of these words will reinforce negative beliefs over time. These words say, "Well, I know I should do this, but I'm not going to. I don't expect to succeed. I'll try again later." It's time to wise up to your self-talk and stop starting over for good! As you continue reading, you'll uncover ways to effectively use transformative language, and you'll come to recognize how the words you choose play into your emotional state.

An effective approach to changing negative language is using the word *when* instead of *if*, *will* instead of *try*, and *know* instead of *hope*. *When* presumes that something will be done, whereas *if* leaves it to chance. Using *when* helps you to believe mentally and emotionally that you've already done something, and the next step is to live out the physical manifestation of that goal. "*When* I get that promotion..." "*When* I lose the weight..." *When* says that you know with conviction in your heart that a goal has been reached. In the famous words of Denzel Washington, "Say thank you in advance for what you already have!"

I also encourage use of the words *I am*, as in *I am strong, I am courageous, I am joyful, and I am fulfilled.* These transformations in your language can have a tremendous impact on how you perceive your life and how you define yourself. Changing your words may seem like a small, subtle thing to do, but I've seen it radically transform thousands of lives!

You can use transformative language as a tool to identify negative thoughts and put a stop to them. Once you recognize how your words affect your life, you'll hire your seven-foot bouncer to stand guard at the doorway of your mind, allowing only positive thoughts into the party. You will no longer allow negative words to throw you off course, because now you're aware that how you speak to yourself can make or break progress. The most beautiful thing about this is that over time, you can condition yourself to get rid of these negative words altogether and never feel the negative emotions that accompany them ever again!

Through working with clients, I've learned that behaviors and thoughts are consistent with who we believe we are. What standards are you working to live up to: poor, good, great, or outstanding? When you speak as if you've already attained a goal, you'll practice more of the behaviors that will help you reach it without even thinking—the days of internal conflict are over, but you won't become a master overnight. Mastering your emotions is a lifelong process, so trade expectation for appreciation, and practice patience with yourself!

CHAPTER 8

PRINCIPLES OF PHYSICAL MASTERY

When most of us think of the word "fitness," we think of physical fitness, weight lifting, and cardio. However, progression of physical, emotional, mental, and spiritual fitness is the recipe for happiness—we cannot put emphasis on only one area. In my experience, many people will simply look to physical exercise to transform their bodies. Although fitness is important, your overall health is a byproduct of your mental, spiritual, and emotional makeup. The goal of this chapter is to teach you the physical principles of my philosophy.

Moving your body is arguably the most effective way to feel better about yourself. Exercise explodes your physiological response and releases dopamine, endorphins, and a whole chemical concoction of "feel good" chemicals.

The way you move your body largely determines how you feel.

PRINCIPLE #1: FIX YOUR FACE

Before we dive into obvious physical principles like fitness, nutrition, and recovery, I want to address something that can instantly change the way you feel. I recommend that you exercise thirty to sixty minutes per day, three to six days per week, but what should you do when you *aren't* exercising? How you use your body during this time has a large impact on your quality of life.

When a person walks into the room with shoulders slumped over, a frown on their face, and eyes on the floor, what is your immediate thought about their state of being? You'd think they were depressed, sad, or in a bad mood, right? However, when a person walks into the room with their head held high and a smile on their face, and they strut with confidence, what is your immediate thought about this person's state of being? You'd think they were excited, happy, and feeling good!

Physical fitness starts with the way you carry yourself. Motion creates emotion. The most underutilized muscles are the eighty muscles in our faces. Most of us go through life without realizing the impact of a smile, laughter, and positive facial expressions on our moods. The movements of your body (especially your face) determine how you feel. Have you ever tried laughing hysterically and pouting simultaneously? It doesn't work very well!

I wanted to kick off the physical principles of fitness with this topic because it's widely overlooked. Make a commitment to yourself to take inventory of your facial expressions on a daily basis. Find things that make you laugh.

SURROUND YOURSELF WITH PEOPLE WHO MAKE YOU SMILE.

Do things that create happiness intentionally. The majority of your time will *not* be spent in the gym, so always remember to use your physical body to create good vibes 24/7!

Each time you feel a negative emotion, force yourself to smile and hold it for one minute. Repetition is the creator of all skills, and the more you smile, the more you'll become addicted to the feeling it gives you.

PRINCIPLE #2: ONE SHOT, ONE OPPORTUNITY

Your physical body is the only one you'll ever get. Take the following illustration into consideration. What if I told you that you were only going to be allowed to drive one car for the rest of your life, and it's the only one you'll ever own. If this car breaks down or becomes inoperable, you'll have to walk, ride a bike, or take the bus for the rest of your life. Would you take care of it differently than your current vehicle? If you're being honest with yourself, this is a no-brainer. The pain of not having the freedom of a vehicle is far greater than the pain of regular oil changes and routine cleanings. Think about when you've taken your car into the shop for repairs. Didn't it drive you crazy to be without your car for just a few hours? What if you never had a car again?

You don't take care of your car as if it were the last one you'll ever have because you know that's not true. Still, the sad thing is, most of us take better care of our cars than we do our own bodies. Think about it. You'd never put diesel fuel into a car that requires premium, as it would ruin the engine. You've never gone the entire winter without a wash, as it creates rust. It's more likely that you've gone weeks, months, or years without properly fueling and maintaining your physical body. When we don't take care of our bodies appropriately and they break down, we don't just lose our health—we lose *everything.* It's astounding how far out of line our priorities can get, but you're never too far gone or too old to begin taking care of your body.

I'll use the famous words of Eminem, the rapper, to ask you an important question: "If you had one shot, or one opportunity to seize everything you've ever wanted, in one moment, would you capture it or just let it slip?" We have one body for the rest of our lives. If we screw it up, we don't get another one. This is why the projection of pain exercise we did works so well. I want to encourage you again to practice this visualization process, because it puts in perspective how important today is.

DO YOU EVEN REALIZE?

Not moving your body is like never driving your car. Even the most expensive cars in the world will not start if you fail to ignite the engine for two years. Our creator specifically designed our bodies for movement. Do you realize how precious a gift this is? The ability to walk, run, lift, jump, and climb is unique to our species. Yet so many of us perceive moving to be too hard, inconvenient, and "not worth it."

There are millions of people on this planet who don't have the same privilege you do. There are kids in your city, right now, who are sitting in a wheelchair praying to God that we develop a cure for their disease. By and large, we take for granted how special it is to move appropriately. Doesn't that put into perspective whatever excuses you've used to not exercise in the past?

I understand that you may not desire to exercise so vigorously, and I'm not suggesting you have to. Did you know that over 60 percent of Americans don't exercise regularly (three times per week or more)? To make this even worse, the American Heart Association considers *walking* exercise! We have become so lazy as a nation that it's too hard to get up and walk down the street!

Imagine you're in a room full of children with muscular dystrophy, and you have to explain to them why you don't move your body daily. You would tell them all the excuses, stories, and reasons why you don't have time, it's too hard, or you don't feel good. This group of kids would literally chop off their right arms if it meant they could experience exercise for even a year.

I know they would, because I'm heavily involved with the Muscular Dystrophy Association (MDA), and I get a chance to hang out with these kids several times a year. We hate it when people call them "children *suffering* with muscular dystrophy." The truth is, they aren't suffering at all. These kids are happier than the majority of normally functioning adults.

You have one body, and by the grace of God it functions appropriately. Take a step back for a moment to consider your movement patterns. What excuse could you possibly have not to walk down the street? Your body is *your temple* that houses all the beautiful memories and love you experience in your life. I want very badly for you to realize it's important to begin executing this *now*, but you've got to want it more than I do.

My job is to be brutally honest with you. Everything in life is binary. With every decision to sit on the couch or go to the gym, overload on sugar or trade it for a salad, binge-watch Netflix or feed your mind with education, you're creating a longer or a shorter life. In other words, you're choosing to create longevity, or you're slowly dying. Make a commitment right now to never let another day pass without considering the impact of every little decision. After all, small, daily decisions will shape your destiny.

PRINCIPLE #3: TRADE YOUR "SHOULDS" FOR "MUSTS"

Jim Rohn is one of the founding fathers of personal development and life coaching. He is a mentor to Tony Robbins and a great inspiration to me as well. Jim shares an eye-opening concept about "shoulds" vs. "musts" that can drastically change the direction of your workout habits. This simple strategy will leave you never saying "should" again!

How often do we say, "I should"? I should get to the office earlier, I should eat better, I should work out every day, and I should do this or do that. We keep doing that until we "should" all over ourselves.

My advice is to stop "shoulding" and trade the word "should" for "must" in your vocabulary. If we say we *must* eat healthier and *must* work out, it becomes a definition of our true behavior, rather than how it "should" be. As humans, we will always do what's in line with how we've defined ourselves. "Must" is a powerful, transformative word that implies there is no option other than taking massive action toward your goals.

Going back to an earlier example, if one of your parents were deathly ill, and your standard is to be an outstanding son or daughter, what would you say and do? You'd never say, "I should find a way to raise the money to save them." You'd say, "I *must* save them."

This simple replacement of one word in your vocabulary creates an entirely different context for the meaning of your statement. When you *must* do something vs. *should* do it, you cut off any possibility of not completing the action. What we really mean when we say "should" is "I know it's the right thing to do, but I'm not going to do it."

Since you're still reading this book, I know you're loving my crazy strategies for designing your life. Here's another one I've used with my successful clients that works really well.

When you catch yourself saying "I should work out today,"

immediately take your right hand, open your palm, hold your open hand above your head, and repeatedly bop yourself on the skull while you say, "I must work out today. I must work out today. I must work out today!" This must be done with a grinning smile from ear to ear.

I know that sounds silly. But if you keep doing the same things you've always done, you'll never change. If you take inventory of all the "shoulds" in your life and trade those for "musts," by default you'll view life through a different lens.

PRINCIPLE #4: DO WHAT YOU LOVE

Just because I'm the founder of Burn Boot Camp doesn't mean you have to join one of my gyms to experience success. I don't compete with anyone else in the industry (I'm my only competition), and I'm not afraid to send you elsewhere. I strive to provide an amazing experience founded on lasting change, and *most* people who start never stop— hence the name of this book, *Stop Starting Over*.

There's one thing I'm certain about. This will be the only body you ever own. You know that when this body stops functioning, your physical presence is gone from the earth. The daily decision to exercise will be a significant factor in experiencing a life long enough to reach your Perfect Day. We've already established that you'll wake up every day to attack this dream. What more urgency do you need to begin or elevate your workout regimen right now?

The best piece of advice I can give about getting fit is to find something you love and stick with it. One reason Burn Boot Camp is a transformative fitness concept is we are able to attract people who have been stagnant for years. We bring them into an environment where moving their body with other like-minded people is fun, and they feel like they are part of a team. It's something they truly enjoy. I would be lying if I told you 100 percent of the people who try Burn end up joining. They don't. Either they weren't ready to make a change and won't work out anywhere, or they didn't enjoy the process of their trial and want to try something different.

I'm a huge advocate of "dating" gyms, personal trainers, boot camps, or boxing gyms until you find what you enjoy. You can succeed at any of these places, but remember: success without fulfillment is considered failure. I need you to enjoy the process of becoming healthy and happy in order to stop starting over. There are hundreds of options available to you. I suggest you choose the program that answers the question "Do I see myself doing this three to six times per week for the rest of my life?" with a resounding "Hell yes, I do!"

There are plenty of fitness clubs and trainers, and I believe you should try several different options before you make a decision. You'd never marry someone after the first date, would you? You'd most likely go on several dates, maybe fall into a relationship with one of them, and eventually find the one you wanted to marry. Do the same thing with your exercise decisions. Date every gym, personal trainer, and boxing gym in your city before you make a decision to join long term. But do yourself a favor—once you've committed, go all in.

Consistency is key, so it's critical to find something that keeps you motivated. You must enjoy the process of fitness with a routine that doesn't feel like a chore, ultimately boosts internal energy and mental strength, and changes your outward appearance.

You don't even need to join a gym. Fitness is free! If you like getting up and running for thirty minutes in the morning, and that's all you want to do, go for it! But don't do yourself a disservice by closing off other options and thinking that's the only way to reach your goals. There are multiple routes available, so be meticulous in your selection, but give 100 percent effort on all of your dates!

Any trainer can show you how to do a push-up or a proper squat. Your job is to find the right one for you, or the right gym, and show up. Take your time to find what works best, but start moving your body in some way, shape, or form *today*. Maybe you start by going for a walk or jog outside right after you're done with this book. When would "now" be a good time?

PRINCIPLE #5: MOTIVATION VS. DEMOTIVATION

Maybe you're extra-motivated right now because you have a tropical vacation, an anniversary, or a high school reunion coming up. Or, you're simply feeling the pain of not being as healthy as you want to be. Then, you pick up this book, your soul is on fire, and you can't wait to get started. You're feeling super-motivated right now, and I hate to burst your bubble, but it's not going to last.

You crush it for sixty days, and you're looking and feeling good. You go on vacation and take pictures of yourself in your bikini or swimsuit on the very first day. After you capture your fit body on camera, you follow your predetermined game plan of consuming all the food and alcohol your body can handle. Then, you get back home, and it's back to reality—time to work out and eat right again. Enter demotivation.

Motivation ebbs and flows. This is why we've installed the principles of your North Star and Perfect Day. You can be extremely motivated for vacations, the New Year, or a high school reunion, but where does the motivation go after those events? Many people start over again because they never discovered their purpose and quit once they reached their short-term goal.

While developing your new mindset, it's important that you discover how the North Star and your motivation work hand in hand. Short-term motivation will give you spikes in results, but with every action, there's an equal and opposite reaction. A period of demotivation kicks in. You're not enthused anymore.

This moment is why you need to have your North Star somewhere visible at all times. This is why it's vitally important to write it down. Every time you feel demotivated, all you have to do is read your North Star paragraphs back to yourself.

The chart below will depict graphically how this works. Everyone experiences periods of motivation and demotivation. The trick to achieving lasting change is to decrease how long the demotivation periods last, not to get rid of them completely. When your self-awareness meets demotivation, you'll easily trigger the North Star thoughts and quickly regain momentum.

MOTIVATION VS. DEMOTIVATION

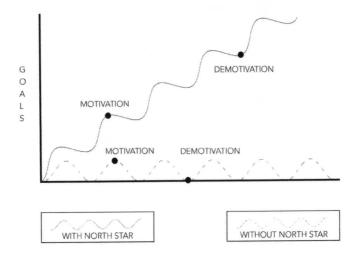

As you can see, with your North Star, you create consistent, long-lasting progress. Without it, you fall into the trap of starting over, again and again. We need to expect failures, setbacks, demotivation, and disappointment, but when you have the correct expectations, you'll be able to appreciate what demotivation does *for* you—not *to* you.

Keep trying and searching until you find what works. When you find it, commit to it. Ensure that the people in your life are aware of your commitment, so they can hold you accountable. Some people like to use a social media channel, like Instagram or Facebook, to make public announcements about their goals. We don't want to let down the people we care about, and announcing goals is a good motivator—we'll gravitate toward actions that make us and others proud. If a trainer or friend feels the satisfaction of our success, it's a victory for everyone!

That being said, never forget that what you do in private shows up in public. Self-accountability is built into the North Star and is the only way to reach your goals. When you learn to stop negotiating with yourself, you'll begin to create the discipline needed to sustain long-term results. Make yourself do what you say you're going to do, when you say you're going to do it. That is the definition of integrity.

PRINCIPLE #6: IT'S YOU VS. YOU

To further encourage you in developing your fitness ritual, I want to emphasize that *you* are your only competition—it's you vs. you, and no one else. Never compare your personal journey to that of others; everyone finds themselves in different circumstances.

Think of the horses in the Kentucky Derby. In addition to their superhero-like masks, they wear blinders to prevent them from looking to their side. They can only see what's in front of them. Why? Because if they focus on the other horses, they will lose a step. When we look at others, we tend to create a false sense of competition that derails our goals. If the horses look left or right, they lose a step. If you are chasing your perceived competition, you aren't chasing your dreams.

With regard to your fitness goals, I encourage you to put blinders on and develop a single-minded focus: to consistently make progress toward your Perfect Day. There will always be somebody out there who's in better shape, but it doesn't matter. All that matters is that you get better every day.

You are beautiful, strong, intelligent, smart, and inspirational in your own way. Nobody else can be you! Take advantage of the uniqueness of who you are and how your higher power has blessed you in life. Let go of the expectations others have for their journey, and appreciate your own!

PRINCIPLE #7: BREAKING DOWN YOUR GOALS

You might be at a peak fitness level while reading this, and you may want to go from 15 to 13 percent body fat. Or maybe you can do ten pull-ups unbroken, and now you want to do twenty. Maybe you want to lose one hundred pounds, but you're fearful of setting the goal, and you have no idea how to reach it. It's most likely your goal is somewhere in the middle of these.

Don't let yourself be paralyzed by huge goals! You can begin your journey to success by putting audacious goals out into the universe. I'm an advocate of dreaming big when others say, "Don't set your goals so high that you are let down when you don't hit them." This is a fantastic mindset to have, and great coaching advice! (That was sarcasm.)

Let's apply reality vs. actuality once again. Is there someone out there who's reached the goal you desire? Of course, there is. Do they have any unique talents, superpowers, or skills you don't have? Of course, they don't. View your goals in the light of actuality, rather than through the reality in the brain today. To make your dreams an actuality, you must create a game plan to tackle your biggest goals.

Let's take a moment to work through a goal backwards and create actionable steps. For example, you want to lose one hundred pounds in twelve months. First, you need to figure out how many pounds per month you need to lose. From there, you break it down even further, into pounds per week, understanding there are 3,500 calories in every pound. What calorie deficit do you need to create on a daily basis to reach that weight loss goal? By drilling down the large task into manageable, daily chunks, you can write the next paragraph or page of your story as you work toward your goal. You have momentum, which creates action, which brings results!

Later in this book, I'll share a story of a client who lost 174 pounds in a year. We broke down her overall goal into smaller daily goals and made them attainable. In her case, she ate 1,800 calories of clean food each day and did one forty-five-minute workout six times per week. The process was manageable, and she had consistent, visible, and motivating results.

Imagine if I said, "Lose one hundred pounds in a year. Ready, go!" What would you think? It sounds difficult, and there's no strategy. If I said, "Eat 1,800 calories and work out for forty-five minutes every day," it's much easier to initiate the belief that you can do it. When you break down lofty goals into manageable chunks, overwhelm is completely removed.

Also, don't let anyone influence how you go about achieving your goals. It might sound like too much to them, and they'll suggest you start with a smaller, ten-pound weight-loss goal. Never let anyone say that you can't aim for the stars! Other people might not be willing to do what it takes to lose the one hundred pounds, but you're different from them. Their advice to you is the advice they would give themselves, and you have higher aspirations. Don't let someone else's standards influence your decision to redefine who you are.

MODELING FOR SUCCESS

An effective tool you can use to achieve success is *modeling*. You know that someone out there has achieved your desired goal before. Muster up the courage to talk to that person, or research them online and find out how they did it. Reverse-engineer those strategies and learning journeys, and adopt them as your own. I can't tell you exactly what to do; I can only explain how to go about it. You may be afraid to ask for help because you don't want to admit you've failed, but the only way you will fail is by continuing to deploy the same strategies. Get a new perspective, and you'll surely gain insights that will help you on your journey!

We all know on an intellectual level that if we work out consistently for thirty to sixty minutes three to six days per week, we will become incrementally more fit. Everyone understands that eating healthily and exercising often are two strategies that can be used in combination to help you reach your fitness goals. Even so, many people talk themselves out of working out before they even get to the gym! Forget about being perfect, and throw away negative principles that get in the way of what you know is right.

PRINCIPLE #8: "DONE FOR YOU" IS "DONE TO YOU"

By now, you know that this book isn't about giving you a ninety-day plan and laying out exactly what to do every step of the way. As the leader of a massive fitness organization, countless trainers, and thousands of clients, I'd be doing you a disservice if I created something that was "done for you." These types of "ninety-day workout plans" are short-term strategies that aren't sustainable. They only focus on the "how to," which is the exact opposite of my philosophy.

If these "how-to" books really work, why are 70 percent of us still overweight? My goal is to mentor you, ask you the right questions, and get you to formulate your own plan. Have you ever heard the Chinese proverb "Give a man a fish and feed him for a day, teach a man to fish and feed him for a lifetime"? The greatest mentors will never give you the answers—they will inspire the right thoughts, so you can create your own plan.

MAKE IT YOURS

As a serial entrepreneur, I oversee large teams of people. I have the privilege of leading in my organizations every day, the biggest one being Burn Boot Camp. As a young leader, I've learned that when *you* make the plan, no one will follow you.

I distinctly remember a time when I faced immense pressure and frustration from business partners, vendors, and clients in Burn's early days. We were growing so fast that our operational capacity couldn't keep pace with our rate of development. The ball was being dropped left and right. I was overwhelmed, and that spilled over to my team, affecting the culture of our brand.

One day, I called a meeting and sat everyone down at a conference table. As I began to lay out all of our problems, the morale in the room dropped quickly. I told them we were implementing an accountability strategy to accelerate our business—we couldn't let anything slip through the cracks. Using a whiteboard, I wrote down the tasks I wanted each person to complete on a weekly basis. Then, I told everyone we would have a meeting at the end of each week to ensure they were doing their jobs correctly.

We carried on this strategy for about three weeks. I noticed our atmosphere and culture had changed, but I didn't know why. In the third week, we had our accountability meeting and I asked each person how they'd done on their weekly project. I've always been intuitive about human behavior, and I picked up on a collective "this is bullshit" frequency from the team.

I immediately stopped what I was doing and said, "You guys hate this, don't you?" My team nodded and shared an overwhelming, collective sigh of relief, as I quickly erased the whiteboard to signify that I agreed.

What happened next was an incredible revelation for me. I asked, "Why didn't you guys tell me you felt this way?" One by one, they laid their feelings out and said it made them feel micromanaged and controlled, and they shared what they thought would fix our problems as an organization. Their plan was *way* better than mine! Not only did they accomplish the outcome of tightening our business up, they also had ideas I never would have come up with on my own!

That day, the *true* leader in me was born. I realized that by asking them a simple question—"Why didn't you guys tell me you felt this way?"—I opened up the door for them to take ownership of their plan for success.

Why am I telling you this story? I made a commitment to myself that day to never bark out orders again. I decided that my standard was no longer to be a good business owner—I wanted to be an outstanding leader.

Imagine being told what to do and when to do it 100 percent of the time in your job. Zero autonomy, no creative stimulus, and a lack of self-confidence would cause you to quit in a heartbeat! So, my question to you is this: how is your fitness journey any different?

Telling you the plan will never help you achieve long-term happiness and success. Focusing on the strategies before focusing on your North Star will have you starting over repeatedly. I strongly believe that leaders, authors, and speakers who have "done for you" strategies are actually creating a false hope that is "done to you."

After years of applicable experience, I can tell you with absolute certainty that the only way you'll create lasting change is when the plan belongs to *you*. I can't and won't tell you what it should be, but I'll offer mentorship and guiding principles along the way.

PRINCIPLE #9: THE POWER OF GROUPING

The strategies to a physically fit life are simple.

1. Move your body three to six times per week for thirty to sixty minutes.
2. Eat whole foods from natural plant sources, but not too much!
3. Feed your mind for thirty to sixty minutes per day.

Most of us create a scenario of 1,000 things we must do to take our fitness to the next level. Have you or someone you know ever been a victim of overcomplicating a fitness strategy so much that it creates snowballing fears and results in zero action? Some people are paralyzed by the fear of doing something new because there is so much in front of them, and it's overwhelming. They don't know where to start, so it's easier to do nothing at all. Read the inner dialogue below and see if it seems familiar.

I should work out more. I should find a gym. Ugh, I hate gyms. That means I have to go online. I'm at work, and I'm not allowed to surf the web. Ugh, I hate work. That means I'll have to do my research during my lunch break and won't have time to eat.

Holy cow, there are twenty gyms in this area alone! How will I choose one? Now I should look up all their numbers and call them. Ugh, I hate calling. I bet they won't answer. But if they do, they will probably try to sell me on a membership. I'll have to take a tour and decide which one I like best. All of them probably charge a lot. Ugh, I hate salespeople.

If I do join one, I guess I'll have to change clothes at work. Then, I'll have to get in my car, put it in reverse and get out of the parking lot. It's so crowded, it will take me five minutes just to get out. Ugh, I hate parking lots. Then, I'll have to park in the back of the gym's parking lot and walk all the way in. I bet all the treadmills will be full. Ugh, I hate running. Oh, man, then I'll be sweaty, and I'll end up having to shower in the locker room. Their locker rooms are gross. This sounds way too complicated. I think I'm going to sit here and eat this pizza.

Humans make everything so damn complicated! We can completely eliminate all this self-inflicted, paralyzing dialogue just by getting up early, putting on our shoes, and running down the street.

The above is a common refrain that *discourages* fitness, and it doesn't have to be that way. We have to stop making this a bigger deal than it is! Make it simple: go to the gym, and work out. Don't feel like going the gym route? Start with something comfortable. Go outside and run or walk. Do push-ups and bodyweight squats in your living room. Go to my YouTube channel and work out with me for free (YouTube.com/DevanKline). Don't worry if you have no idea what you're doing—I'll coach you through it!

When you add a thousand steps to a simple process, the phrase "one, two, three steps...too many" becomes relevant, and the brain creates complication. If there seem to be more than just a few things to be done to get somewhere, the majority of us won't do them, because the likelihood of failure increases. We tend to overthink and interject uncertainty, which paralyzes action.

You don't have to spend hours researching gyms or trainers. Focus on one action—reaching your North Star—and take simple, effective steps to get there. Physical fitness *must* become part of your life, and it's not complicated!

BURST TRAINING (MY PERSONAL FAVORITE STYLE)

You don't have to train for two hours per day to become a physically fit person. For busy people who struggle to find time to work out during the day, I'd like to recommend my go-to strategy. It's minimal, effective, and put me on the map as a personal trainer. Welcome to Burst Training!

Burst Training is a fifteen-minute period each day where you choose five body-weight strength and conditioning exercises. These incorporate the upper and lower body, the core, agility work, and cardio. Each intense exercise is performed for twenty seconds, followed by twenty seconds of *active rest*, which brings the intensity down without stopping—you can hop in place in what I call a "boxer stance."

The goal of Burst Training is to get your heart rate to 90 percent of maximum in twenty seconds and then allow it to come down to 60 percent during the rest periods. This creates a scientific "afterburn" effect in your body that dramatically increases your metabolism and levels of HGH, testosterone, estrogen, and leptin, while decreasing cortisol, the stress hormone. Burst Training is also extremely effective—it's proven to burn an average of nine times more calories than a thirty-minute treadmill run!*

Another reason why Burst Training is awesome is that you can do it any time, any place, and you don't need equipment—you use your body weight! Your body is your barbell, and fifteen minutes a day is all it takes to create a wealth of positive emotion, strength, energy, and vitality. Energy gained from physical movement allows you to create, learn, and imagine more, and pass those positives along to your family and loved ones.

If the thought of working out in your office or living room or outside during your lunch break isn't motivating, I still encourage you to give it a shot. If you've never worked out before, I don't recommend doing this six days a week to start. Begin with fifteen minutes, three days a week, and once you are ready to increase the frequency, you can join me on my YouTube channel for absolutely no cost. I add new workouts each week!

---

* Pete McCall, "7 Things to Know about Excess Post-Exercise Oxygen Consumption (EPOC)," American Council on Exercise, Aug. 24, 2014, https://www.acefitness.org/education-and-resources/professional/expert-articles/5008/7-things-to-know-about-excess-post-exercise-oxygen-consumption-epoc.

★ CHAPTER 9 ★

NUTRITION

The food we eat is made up of calories, which are units of energy for the human body. Along with oxygen, it's what keeps our bodies functioning. Every calorie is composed of three macronutrients called proteins, fats, and carbohydrates. These units of energy we put into our bodies determine our internal health and play a role in our body composition. Most of us understand how vital nutrition is to our overall well-being, but over 70 percent of our society is still overweight.

According to a study done by the radio program *Marketplace*, 70 percent of the American diet consists of processed food.* *Pandora's Lunchbox* author Melanie Warner says the processed-food revolution began over

---

* Kai Ryssdal, "Processed Foods Make up 70 Percent of the American Diet," *Marketplace*, March 12, 2013, https://www.marketplace.org/2013/03/12/life/big-book/processed-foods-make-70-percent-us-diet.

one hundred years ago and has gradually continued to take over the American diet. Warner says that there are an estimated 5,000 different additives allowed to go into our food, but:

> The FDA doesn't actually know how many additives are going into our food. This is in part because regulations are not only self-regulatory—so the food industry is doing the testing—but it's also voluntary. The ingredient companies don't actually have to tell the FDA about a new ingredient. If they choose to, they can simply just launch it into the market. The FDA doesn't know about them, and nobody else really knows about them.

The entire nutritional system is a mess, but you don't have to be a part of it. Just like everything else in life, it's your choice to practice outstanding nutritional habits. Wouldn't it be nice to no longer feel imprisoned by food? Let's dive into the psychology around nutrition and get you eating clean by default.

PRINCIPLE #1: RECOGNIZE THE ACTUAL PROBLEM

Big American food companies seem to care about only one thing: money. They put ingredients in our food that are banned in other countries. Could it be that these ingredients are leading to a drastically unhealthy nation? The Institute of Medicine and National Research Council report that Americans are "sicker and die younger" than people in other wealthy nations.[*] When compared to sixteen other wealthy nations, the US ranks last in overall health and life expectancy. This is sad, considering we spend 2.5 times more on healthcare than any other nation.[†] Our health seems to be the least of concerns to these food companies. In fact, the goal of becoming a healthier population is detrimental to their business goals.

I've followed food blogger and *New York Times* best-selling author Vani Hari, more commonly known as "Food Babe," for several years. Hari is a leading food activist and has created a lot of noise surrounding "Big Food" companies and their role in these eye-opening health statistics. Hari's campaigns are said to be responsible for influencing companies like Kraft and Chick-fil-A to make major changes in their ingredient lineup.

Hari writes, "The victims of obesity are likely the same victims of systematic brainwashing from Big Food marketers, relying on diet soda or low fat products, or looking

[*] Sarah Boseley, "Americans Are 'Sicker and Die Younger' Than People in Other Wealthy Nations," *The Guardian*, Jan. 10, 2013, https://www.theguardian.com/world/2013/jan/10/americans-sicker-die-younger.

[†] Richard Knox, "US Ranks below 16 Other Rich Countries in Health Report," NPR, Jan. 9, 2013, https://www.npr.org/sections/health-shots/2013/01/09/168976602/u-s-ranks-below-16-other-rich-countries-in-health-report.

only at calories on product labels. Basically, they are doing what the food industry has been teaching them about losing weight versus finding out the truth about real food."

With Big Food companies leading discussion and education surrounding food and nutrition, it's no surprise that the masses are blind to making healthy decisions. "Unfortunately, the doctors in this country are not exactly leading the discussion either, since nutrition is not currently a focus in medical school. And the government has their hands tied by big food industry and chemical company lobbyists that basically control what the FDA approves, deems safe for human consumption, and our overall food policy," writes Hari. Big industries and the medical model aren't keen to change, because their pockets would be significantly impacted.

Don't count on a significant change to the American food system anytime soon. It's our job to get educated about what's really in our food and take control of what we put into our bodies. We can no longer allow these food companies to persuade us to buy "healthy choices" with their clever marketing.

THE REAL ENEMY

The traditional medical model is clearly failing us. We are conditioned to think pills will fix our ailments. Why? Again, because Big Food and Medicine control marketing—the vehicle by which we receive our information. We only know what we are exposed to. I want to introduce you to an alternative to the traditional medical model called *functional medicine.*

Functional medicine is a combination of bioavailable nutrients focused on creating optimal functioning of the body and its organs. Functional medicine has one drug: food. The biggest driver of disease is inflammation, and the modern-day diet is full of inflammatory foods like processed sugar, hydrogenated oils, vegetable oil, fatty meats, whole and 2 percent milk, cheese, sugary yogurt, white bread, and fast foods. Inflammation promotes an environment in the body where disease can thrive. Nutrition isn't about losing weight—it's about creating alkalinity in the body (the opposite of acidity), and weight loss is the byproduct of a normal-functioning ecosystem.

THE ENEMY ISN'T CARBS, SUGARS, OR FATS.

They don't make human beings fat and sick; the real enemy is *acidity.* Big Food corporate marketing hangs its unique selling points on low-carb, low-sugar, and low-fat items to entice you to pull the trigger and choose its product over the competitor's. What the ads don't tell you is that the artificial ingredients used to replace your real nutrients aren't really nutrients at all.

Your brainpower, energy levels, appearance of your skin, and vitality are all optimized by properly nourishing your body. Food is such a powerful thing! It's not "normal" to have headaches, gas, gut pain, and acidic reactions from food. This might be hard to comprehend, because we see coughing, sneezing, and having the flu as the norm. These ailments are self-induced, and it's not our fault—it's the byproduct of the Big Food and Medical companies leading us down a path to consume allogeneic, inflammatory, and toxic foods that create acidity in our bodies.

Food is the regulator of your physiology, and it's not normal to feel "fine." Most days, you should feel great. When we defined our standards earlier in the book, which one did you choose? Poor, good, great, or outstanding? When your standards are outstanding, you create a maximized quality of life for yourself and for those around you. How can you possibly have the energy to live life at a high level when you're routinely putting toxic foods and chemicals into your system? You wouldn't put diesel fuel into your Lambo, would you?

Have you ever heard of the "frog in the water" metaphor? When you place a frog in a boiling pot of water, it will immediately jump out. On the other hand, when you place a frog into cold water and gradually turn up the heat, it will boil to death.

This is exactly what is happening with our food consumption. We consume toxicity in small amounts every day, and over time it builds up and creates an acidic environment—one that allows deadly disease to thrive and take over our bodies.

Everything in life is binary, and our pH balance is no different. Our bodies are always either slightly alkaline or slightly acidic. Foods create an acidic environment or an alkaline one; there's no in-between. Think of cookies, candy, cooking oils, meat, fast food, soda, and processed sugars as the most common acidic foods. On the other hand, avocados, green vegetables, and quinoa help create alkalinity.

On the pH scale, humans should ideally be slightly alkaline, at about 7.18 to 7.2. You can purchase pH strips at any pharmacy to test your alkalinity. Through trial and error, you can work on further understanding alkaline balance and make the conscious decision to control your inputs.

PRINCIPLE #2: THE SIMPLE STRATEGY

Wouldn't it be great to never spend money on pills again, get rid of chronic headaches, be free from the flu, and thrive every single day? The decision to eat the right foods may be difficult, but knowing which foods to eat to create an alkaline environment is simple!

Creating health is about what you do *most of the time*. Just as you'll become what you think about most of the time, what you eat most of the time influences how you'll physically feel. I've included a chart of alkaline vs. acidic foods. Choose from the left side of the chart most of the time, and you will build alkalinity that gives you unlimited amounts of energy and mental clarity. If you choose foods from the right side most of the time, it will result in poor energy, sickness, excess body fat, and a perfect environment for disease to thrive.

I want to open you up to choices, not take them away. My job isn't to tell you what to do, but rather educate you on what the ultimate result of your nutritional choices will be. "Living it up" because life is short is a bad strategy. Life is long, and our lives are a culmination of the choices we make every day.

ALKALINE

- grasses
- cucumber
- Himalayan salt
- kale
- kelp
- spinach
- broccoli
- sprouted beans
- avocado
- beet root
- basil
- collard greens
- ginger
- lettuce
- mustard greens
- okra
- onion
- tomato
- lemons and limes
- butter beans
- soy beans
- chia seeds
- quinoa
- coconut
- watercress
- grapefruit
- pomegranate
- buckwheat
- tofu
- lentils
- rhubarb
- celery
- goat milk
- almond milk
- avocado, olive, coconut, flax oil
- carrot
- cauliflower
- new potatoes
- leeks
- peas
- arugula
- artichokes
- asparagus
- brussels sprouts
- zucchini

ACIDIC

- black beans
- chickpeas
- kidney beans
- seitan
- cantaloupe
- fresh dates
- nectarines, plums
- sweet cherries
- watermelon
- mint
- oats
- spelt
- couscous
- brown rice
- freshwater wild fish
- rice milk
- soy milk
- brazil nuts
- ketchup
- mayonnaise
- butter
- apples
- bananas
- strawberries
- vegan cheese
- rye bread
- wild rice
- alcohol
- coffee
- honey
- jam, jelly
- mustard
- soy sauce
- eggs
- dairy milk
- pecans
- hazelnuts
- wholemeal bread
- vinegar
- yeast
- beef
- chicken
- shellfish
- artificial sweeteners
- blueberries
- mushrooms

COMMON INGREDIENTS TO AVOID

Artificial Colors
- Blue 1, Blue 2, Green 3, Orange B, Citrus Red 2, Yellow 5, Yellow 6, Yellow 10, Red 10, Red 4, Red 3, Red 40

Artificial Sweeteners
- Acesulfam-K, Aspartame, Cyclamates, Saccharin, Stevia, Sucralose, Neotame

Preservatives
- TBHQ, Polysorbates 60, 65, & 80, BHT/BHA, Sodium Benzoate, Sulfites

Artificial Flavors
- Diacetyl, Isoamyl Acetate, Benzaldehyde, Cinnamic Aldehyde, Ethyl Proprionate, Methyl Anthranilate, Limonene, Ethyl Decadienoate, Allyl Hexonate, Ethyl Maltol, Ethylvanillin, Methyl Salicylate

High-Fructose Corn Syrup

Trans Fats

Monosodium Glutamate (MSG)

PRINCIPLE #3: REMOVING TEMPTATION

One of the easiest ways to practice outstanding nutrition is to remove the temptation. But right now, I want to address willpower. Have you ever heard someone say, "I just need more willpower, and I would eat better!" Let's take a look at willpower and see how effective a strategy it really is.

What's your vice? Think of the food you know you're not supposed to eat but you do anyway—I want you to get the picture of that food in your head. Okay, now imagine mountains of this food on a table sitting in the middle of an empty room. You are locked in this room for twenty-four hours with no access to any other food. Now imagine you are forced to walk around this table staring at this food, smelling it, and practically tasting how delicious it is for an entire twenty-four-hour period.

The first hour is no problem. You're convinced that you aren't going to eat this food. By lunchtime, you grow hungry and the food starts to smell even better. By midafternoon you can't think about anything but food. By dinnertime, what will most likely happen? That whole mountain of food overwhelms your senses, and you dive in and binge until only crumbs are left.

I understand this isn't a realistic scenario, but isn't this what we do when we "diet"? You make a decision to eat salads, drink water, and eliminate sugar and alcohol. You start off the week with two solid days of following the rules. By day three, you are feeling good about your progress and start to sneak in little snacks here and there. By Friday night, you convince yourself that you've done well and a little bread won't hurt. By Sunday, you've had a full-blown relapse, only to become disgusted with yourself enough find motivation for the next week.

Willpower is bullshit, and it doesn't work. What you're really searching for is *discipline*. Where does discipline come from? A healthy dose of your North Star, with a side of your Perfect Day, and a sprinkle of self-awareness every day.

You know that if you circle a table of your favorite foods for twenty-four hours, you'll give in. This doesn't make you weak. The important element of discipline is to understand your own triggers and reduce the amount of stimulus you receive from them.

If you've had a pattern of walking into the grocery store past the doughnut aisle and have been unable to resist doughnuts, have the discipline to remove that habit. Go to a different grocery store, or order your groceries online. If you pass the same fast food restaurant on your way home and make frequent stops out of impulse, try a different route home. Removing the temptation is a great way to reduce the amount of times you give in.

WHO IS IN CHARGE?

I've trained a lot of mothers in my career, and I've learned that mothers tend to snack on their kids' food. You may not believe me or even want to hear this, but *you* control what they eat. It's your choice to bring Goldfish and graham crackers into the house. Saying "my kid won't eat anything else" is a cop out for your lack of patience. If you allow them to eat these things, you condition them to want more, and it will become harder to get their buy-in to healthy food. Are you parenting your kids, or are they parenting you? My children have been dairy-, gluten-, and grain-free since birth, and they don't know any different. Remember our ownership talk? If you want to change, you can no longer point the blame at anyone else for your own lack of discipline, especially your children.

With that being said, don't expect to be perfect, as perfection is the ultimate failure. Health is determined by what you eat most of the time, not all of the time. Give them treats, but don't keep them in the house. Discipline is like a muscle. The more times you flex it, the stronger it will become. The more times you successfully remove temptation, the more confidence you will build.

PRINCIPLE #4: INTERRUPT YOUR PATTERNS

If you know what to eat and still don't eat it, you're stuck in an unhealthy pattern. Over the past six years, I've studied neuro-linguistic programming (NLP). First created in the 1970s by Richard Bandler and John Grinder, this approach draws connections among neurological processes (*neuro-*), language (*linguistic*), and behavioral patterns learned through experience (*programming*). Understanding and changing these links can help us set and achieve important life goals. While the practice of NLP is quite complex, the application to changing your behavior patterns is quite simple. Before we dive into how to use NLP to change your eating behaviors, I want to assure you that this will not be an overload of neuroscience. My goal is to give you practical ways to use NLP, not to show you how smart I am.

Have you ever heard of "pattern interrupts" or "breaking patterns"? To achieve this, we must consciously identify the negative behavior we want to eliminate, replace it with a positive behavior, and positively reinforce those actions. This requires a clear self-awareness of what negative behaviors you need to change so that you can identify them and kick this strategy into gear!

Let's get practical.

You will always have a trigger. Whether you're sitting on the couch, driving in your car, working on a project, or stressed out by kids, an event always precedes your behavior. The urge to eat comes about because of this event. Then, we usually walk mindlessly to the pantry and grab acidic food without thinking of its long-term negative effects.

This is where self-awareness must kick in. When you open the pantry and see a big ol' box of cookies, take a moment and ask yourself, "Do these cookies align with my goals?" If the answer is "no," you must immediately do something drastically different.

For example, you could laugh out loud hysterically at yourself and repeat, "I'm not hungry! *The* brain is hungry, not me! This is hilarious!" You can do this to break the pattern of "see food, eat food." Immediately after this pattern is broken, you must do something you enjoy that replaces it. You could reach for some fruit, drop down and do push-ups, listen to your favorite song, dance like crazy, or sing at the top of your lungs. I know this sounds silly, but isn't trying the same strategy over and over insane? Would you rather be silly, or insane?

Next, you want to reinforce this pattern with love and positivity. As humans, we all share the need for love, so love on yourself for a moment! Hug yourself, give yourself a high five, pat yourself on the back, or kiss yourself in the mirror! The last step is to repeat, out loud, "YES! YES! YES!" twenty times in a row, at the top of your lungs. This will force you to smile, and the positivity will reinforce the pattern you just broke by creating a new neuro-association to the food you just ate—you'll disengage from the old behavior. It's important to be LOUD so that your central nervous system (CNS) is conditioned to feel the positivity.

So, let me sum up this strategy. It's taken me six years to master what I am about to tell you in four lines.

1. Notice the undesired behavior.
2. Replace it with a desirable behavior.
3. Reinforce the desirable behavior with self-love.
4. Ingrain the self-love into your CNS vocally.

I told you I was going to give you choices, and here they are. After you break your pattern and eat the handful of grapes, you can still have a cookie if you really want one! But chances are that you feel good about overcoming the temptation, so your brain associates *not* eating the cookies with a pleasurable experience. This weakens the neuro-association of cookies and happiness.

Everything boils down to pain or pleasure, and you can use both to your advantage when you understand psychology. Cookies brought you pleasure in the past, but the grapes will slowly become your default response next time you feel a *real* hunger cue. You didn't build a strong association with bad eating patterns overnight, so practice patience when getting rid of it.

REAL VS. FALSE CUES

Sometimes you are hungry, and other times you *think* you're hungry. Think about a time when you said, "I'm starving," and then received an important text message or phone call. What happened? Your new focus took you away from the thought of eating, and you began to focus on this important conversation. Before you know it, you've completed the call, and you don't feel the urge to eat anymore. Sound familiar? That's because it was a false hunger cue. Be on the lookout for these! If your pattern doesn't naturally get interrupted by a phone call, you may want to consider some type of physical activity to break your pattern. You'll know you're getting a *real* cue when your stomach gurgles or you feel a slight energy drop. This is the perfect time to use healthy food to replace the pattern of toxic food!

PRINCIPLE #5: DON'T LET THE WEEKEND BE YOUR WEAK END

When making the choice to eat better, you must understand your options and the potential result of each one. You have the option to grab a cookie or a cluster of grapes. You have the option to drink a second beer. But you also have the opportunity to create health. Many people have good intentions and attempt to balance healthy eating with their social lives, but it becomes an "all-in or all-out" cycle. They eat loads of toxic food, chase it with alcohol, and end up five pounds heavier the next day. On Monday, they begin to eat clean again and continue that for four days. Then, the weekend hits, and they eat toxic food again.

DO YOU REALIZE THAT THE WEEKEND MAKES UP 28.5 PERCENT OF YOUR ENTIRE WEEK? DON'T LET THE WEEKEND BE YOUR WEAK END.

If you're putting toxicity into your body more than a quarter of the time, will you create alkalinity or acidity? Will repeating that cycle of toxicity lead you to your North Star? Is it even possible to have maximized quality of life if you are overweight, lethargic, or sick? I'm promoting a paradigm shift in this book. I don't need you to be "all-in or all-out" all the time. I need you to look at your lifestyle and make your daily decisions based on *what* you want and *why* you want it, with a focus on the long term.

I'm not saying never go out with friends and never drink wine or eat steak, but let your outstanding standards dictate your choices. Have a salad on the side, or put the steak in it. Drink wine before dinner and lemon water with your meal. You can have a cookie, but choose to eat fruit more often. By consistently eating in this fashion, you'll never have to count calories or struggle with weight ever again. Acidic food will most likely creep into your diet. When it does, I challenge you to couple it with alkaline foods to balance your health.

PRINCIPLE #6: FIVE TRAVEL RULES

Travel is inevitable for some of us. I don't mean vacation;

I mean routine travel for work. My good friend and sports journalist Shannon Spake says, "You're not on a vacation when you travel for work." So here are a few tips to help you on the road.

1. **Eat mono meals.** Eating only one type of food at a particular sitting is called a *mono meal*. For example, stop at Hudson News in the airport and buy four bananas for a meal. Your body easily identifies with one nutritional matrix and can break down and absorb the food much easier. I travel often and have been able to maintain my target fitness levels because of this strategy. This strategy satisfies my nutritional needs and gives me the confidence to eat healthily anywhere.

2. **Pack dry goods.** In mono meal fashion, bring a bag of almonds, cashews, and dried cranberries with you. You can get these foods through airport security, and they can hold you over until you land. I've even been known to throw in some dark chocolate for a little balance.

3. **Pack vitamins and protein powder.** Shaklee Vitalizer is my go-to, and it keeps my energy high. This is my functional medicine in a portable mini-strip. I also use a variation of protein powders on the road. One is a meal replacement powder called Shaklee Life—with a balance of macros, vitamins, and minerals—as well as Afterburn by Burn Nutrition for post-workout. You can take as much as you want through security—there's no hassle!

4. **Find hot bars or buffets.** When you land, chances are you'll have a hot bar or buffet near you. You may have to drive fifteen minutes out of the way to go to Whole Foods, but more often than not, you'll have the option. At the very least, stop at a normal grocery store and get another mono meal.

5. **You can eat healthily anywhere.** My fitness clients often tell me, "I have to wine and dine my prospects to make the sale." Okay, I won't argue that having a few drinks may help you loosen up, but keep in mind that tequila is lowest on the glycemic index, so drink smart! Trade IPAs for a shot mixed with water. Your choice of entrée definitely won't influence the sale. You won't lose a client because you ordered the California salad for dinner, I promise. If you do choose alcohol, never couple it with a poor meal.

PRINCIPLE #7: FIVE VACATION RULES

A vacation is different from travel—it's a time to relax and treat yourself. While vacations are wonderful, they can't be used as an excuse to go overboard with the indulgences, or to ditch your North Star. Take these five rules with you, so you won't stray from the path to success!

1. **Don't sell your home.** You know you're coming back to your house even if you go to the Bahamas for a week, right? Just because you go on vacation doesn't mean

you're selling your home. Meaning: just because you plan to modify a healthy diet while you're gone, don't "sell away" your rituals. You'll stray from your normal routine, but have a game plan ready for when you return home. Don't let your one-week vacation turn into six months of poor choices.

2. **Move every day.** You're going to consume extra calories, so make it a point to exercise for at least fifteen minutes every day. You can use my YouTube videos to exercise with me anywhere in the world.

3. **Follow the three-for-one rule.** For every meal you eat that doesn't align with your North Star, eat three meals that do. It's okay to go on vacation knowing you're going to modify your health path, but completely blowing it up will leave you unfulfilled. Remember: you're always coming back home. Having a good time shouldn't be linked to pigging out on food. If anything, use your vacation as a time to eat premium foods you normally wouldn't have access to, especially if you're near the ocean.

4. **Drink lemon water all day long.** I strongly believe that lemons in your water must be an everyday habit, but especially when you're on vacation. We tend to overload toxicity on vacation, and consuming liquid alkalinity will combat its negative effects.

5. **Plan to start a cleanse the moment you get home.** Have a healthy cleanse waiting for you when you get home. Plan to do Shaklee's Healthy Cleanse or a

steady diet of fruits and vegetables for three to seven days. You can reverse the harm done on vacation with a simple decision to detox. The trick to detoxing is not to "retox." In other words, don't detox for seven days and then feel so accomplished that you pig out upon its completion.

PRINCIPLE #8: FIVE AT-HOME RULES

It's simple to establish at-home rules and rituals, because we are there the majority of the time. Use these five rules to navigate your nutrition rituals while at home!

1. **Follow the twelve-hour rule.** Modify your healthy lifestyle for twelve hours each week. This is not optional. You can't go "all-in" all the time. Go out to eat with your spouse, have a girls' night, or take your kids to breakfast and eat pancakes. You get twelve *consecutive hours* per week to allow less-than-outstanding nutrition into your body. This is not long enough to form a habit, and not short enough to get FOMO (fear of missing out). This integration has been vital to the health of my clients.

2. **Create hydration events.** I want you to commit to drinking roughly half your body weight in ounces of water every day. Squeeze half a lemon into two hydration "events." This is a simple strategy that forces you to set aside five minutes two times per

day to focus only on drinking as much water as you can. This will eliminate forgetting to drink water due to a busy schedule. Adding freshly squeezed lemon to your water creates a constant input of alkalinity. Hydrating your body properly keeps you mentally sharp so that you can discern the real hunger cues from the false ones.

3. **Exercise three to six times, for thirty to sixty minutes each time.** If you don't have ninety minutes per week to exercise, you don't have a life. Time and time again, exercise has been proven to be a more effective antidepressant than Prozac. You will be more likely to practice outstanding nutrition habits when coupled with effort in the gym.

4. **Take a multivitamin.** Strategically planned meals and focused hydration are a great start, but you still won't get everything you need—supplements can provide you with all the nutrients your body requires. Five years ago, I began taking Shaklee's Vitalizer, and since then, I've become affiliated with the organization. It was the first company to create the multivitamin, and it does more than 300 contaminant tests on every ingredient it uses. Nearly 100 percent of supplements on retail shelves are riddled with chemicals, fake ingredients, fillers, and additives. Since they are not regulated or tested by the FDA, standards are low, and there is no guarantee of what's really in the bottle. Shaklee goes above and beyond when it comes to purity and

quality, and that's why I'm such a big proponent of the organization. We carry their products at all Burn Boot Camps, my family uses them, and many of my clients do, as well. I highly recommend the Vitalizer.

5. **Schedule time for meal prep.** Designate one day per week as your meal-prep day. Set aside two hours on that day for meal preparation. Schedule the day and stick to it. Set a reminder on your phone if needed, or make it a weekly family activity. Choose nine foods you enjoy eating that align with your goals—the ones that give you energy and nourish your body. You'll divide these nine foods into categories: three proteins, three carbs, and three fruits or vegetables. You'll also need twelve twenty-four-ounce plastic or glass containers.

★ I recommend Sunday nights for meal prep, since that's usually the most relaxed time of the week. Everything from the previous week is done, and you're preparing for the next one, anyway, so this fits right in. Use whatever cooking device you'd like: a grill, oven, Crock-Pot, or pressure cooker—my favorite is the InstaPot.

★ You'll cook three foods from each category. Let's say the proteins are organic chicken breasts, ground turkey, and grass-fed beef. Make three four- to six-ounce servings of each. Do the same with the carbs as well as fruits and vegetables. Once everything is cooked or prepared, make twelve meals by separating the foods into the twenty-four-ounce containers. Fill each container with one portion of each food type. Mix and match whatever you feel will go well together, and be sure each container is full enough that you can't see the bottom.

★ Instead of counting calories all week, you'll eat two or three of these meals each day, over a five-day period. This plan allows you to stay on track with your goals. Before you leave in the morning, grab the meals and put them in your bag. Oftentimes when we get hungry, we don't have easily accessible food, and we end up eating junk or at the cafeteria buffet at work. This plan gives you better options. You can still go out to lunch with coworkers or grab something from the buffet, but the meal-prep routine provides you with convenient, healthy options. You're feeding your body live-enzyme foods, and if you happen to eat something with high toxicity, there's a fruit or vegetable nearby to counteract the acidity.

THE FIT PACK

To meet your fitness goals and get everything you want from your body, I encourage you to take Shaklee's Performance Fitness Pack, in addition to drinking its smoothies. This is a package of four supplements that help build muscle, increase energy, hydrate, and recover from exercise. I had the privilege of working closely with Shaklee's innovation team at the California headquarters to develop a fitness supplement line, which included the Fit Pack.

The Fit Pack incorporates a whey protein called Build. It's low in carbohydrates and sugar, and it includes a pre-workout energy supplement. It contains another supplement proven to hydrate better than water, as well as a recovery pill made from highly concentrated elements of tart cherry. In my personal case studies and in many of my clients' reports, the Fit Pack has helped them train harder and longer, see better results, and feel great about themselves.

ARE YOU READY?

Are you ready to start fueling your body? I can't tell you what to do; I can only ask you the right questions so that you can formulate your own plan. Are you ready to start eating to live and not living to eat? Eating is a ritual in itself—we must eat to survive. The question is, are you eating to survive, or to thrive? In either case, your energy outputs will directly correlate with your nutritional rituals. We eat food, but we need to view it as more than that— we need to see it as nourishment for our life. There has to be a strategy to your energy. It takes energy to reach your North Star, and you want the most efficient energy possible. The energy resource inside of you is unlocked and released through proper nourishment.

Proper nourishment doesn't have to be a grandiose goal. You don't have to exhaustively research organic foods, wander around the grocery store wondering what to buy, or drown in waves of contradictory nutrition blogs. Stop kidding yourself. You know what to do, and the strategies aren't complex. Eat foods that come from the earth, and don't overeat.

We've discussed that inputs equal outputs when it comes to food and daily activity. Twinkies and pizza will not produce a healthy body, just as binge-watching reality TV will not stimulate you intellectually. Inputs that don't align with your North Star won't provide you with the energy to play with your kids after a long day at work or start that new business—garbage in equals garbage out.

PRINCIPLE #9: NEW DIETS ARE OLD NEWS

The keto, Atkins, and Mediterranean diets as well as intermittent fasting, carb cycling, and virtually every other diet fad that exists are a root cause of the obesity problem, because they are used improperly. I don't recommend diets that cause a symptom lineup similar to many over-the-counter drugs, and I don't recommend them to any clients. These diets are just more "quick-weight-loss" trends, much like the Atkins Diet, which has been criticized for its negative effects on the metabolism. Our society goes crazy over new diets because they are unwilling to address the real problem. These fads are strategy overload and give people false hopes of succeeding long-term. Food exists to nourish your body and cure ailments, not create them. Have you ever seen the list of potential side effects from a keto diet?

★ Constipation
★ Diarrhea
★ Hypoglycemia
★ Frequent urination
★ Drowsiness or dizziness
★ Muscle cramps
★ Sugar cravings
★ Flu-like symptoms (aka "keto flu")
★ Sleep problems
★ "Keto breath"
★ Heart palpitations
★ Reduced strength and physical performance

There's no doubt you can lose weight on the keto diet, but you can do the same by eating a well-balanced diet. Losing weight is about creating a caloric deficit, meaning the energy coming into your body is slightly lower than the energy going out. This scientific fact about human beings has been understood for hundreds of years. None of these diets will work if a human being eats 10,000 calories per day, even if it's clean food.

Most of us are curious about these diets because we want to lose the weight overnight. If you're a bodybuilder approaching a competition, this may be appropriate because specialty diets can target body fat, but I don't recommend rapid weight loss for the average person. If a diet like intermittent fasting is part of your lifestyle, I wouldn't balk at that—just be aware that these diets are advanced, and you must work your way into them. Part of the problem with our society is that we want to focus on strategies and quick results without having a real purpose behind them. My mission is to help create a societal paradigm shift so that we can stop chasing fad diets and start creating lasting change.

Any diet that discourages foods with living enzymes such as fruits, nuts, tubers, and green vegetables is doing a disservice to your long-term health. We've got it all wrong. We immediately think "how to" instead of "why?" We think "short-term quick fix" instead of "long-term rituals."

The keto diet is surely not a lifestyle, and if you're wondering whether you should use it or not, I suggest that you find your purpose for wanting to reach your goals and find something that allows you to look beyond just the next thirty days.

The strategy is simple: your energy intake must be slightly less than energy output. Figure out your total daily energy expenditure (TDEE) at TDEECalculator.net. To lose one pound per week, you'll need to eat 500 calories less than your TDEE per day. Ultimately, building muscle is what will keep the weight off long-term, because muscle burns three times more calories at rest than body fat.

To maintain muscle, you must ensure that your body gets at least half a gram of protein per pound of body weight. If you'd like to build muscle, I suggest increasing your protein intake to one gram per pound. The remainder of your calories should consist of alkaline carbs like quinoa and alkaline fats like avocados.

Use your North Star to figure out your strategies. Losing weight should never be the goal; creating optimal health should be the goal. Through this lens, body-fat loss becomes a byproduct of a healthy lifestyle and consumption of the appropriate amounts of calories with proper nutrients.

★ CHAPTER 10 ★

RECOVERY

Sleep is an extremely important ritual for muscle building and recovery. When we work out, we micro-tear our muscle fibers, causing them temporary damage. The nutrition we put into our bodies along with our sleeping patterns work in combination to allow our bodies to recover. Sleep is one of the most overlooked elements of happiness, especially for entrepreneurs and parents.

Numerous books, podcasts, and entrepreneurial coaches chastise people for sleeping too much and wasting time. There's an element of truth to that if you sleep twelve hours a day. On the flip side, workaholics pontificate on the "benefits" of sleeping four hours a night in order to stay productive. That's bad advice. I'm not worried about what you don't get done while you sleep—I'm concerned with what you do while you're awake. A solid six to eight hours of sleep each night should be your target.

Your body will thank you, and so will your family, friends, and coworkers!

To have vibrant energy during the sixteen hours you are awake, give back, and be your best self, quality sleep is a must! Being well-rested also allows you to pursue fitness goals with verve and have mental clarity to make good choices. After all you've learned, you'd be doing yourself a disservice not to receive the acute mental gift that regular sleeping patterns give you. Personally, I sleep six hours every night. After much trial and error, I discovered the pattern that balances my sleep with the maximum energy I need for the day.

After reading this book, you won't magically walk away with a strategy in place; you'll need to practice different sleeping patterns until you find your groove. Try sleeping six hours one night, and make a note of what your energy is like the next day. Then, try sleeping seven, and then eight. Keep track of how you feel each time. I don't recommend sleeping more than eight hours—it's a waste of time. We don't need ten hours of sleep to rejuvenate the mind, body, and spirit. That six- to eight-hour time frame is the "sweet spot" to dial in daily energy needs for the majority of us.

For example, if you're a marathon runner putting in twelve miles a day, you might need a full eight hours of sleep to recover effectively. If you're a businessperson traveling a great deal and encountering stress on a regular basis, you probably need eight hours to let your cortisol hormones metabolize overnight. As we've learned throughout this book, it's all about finding what works best for you and making the choices that align with your North Star. I can't tell you what to do; I can only teach you the principles and allow you to find the answers. If your Perfect Day has you owning and operating a successful business, then six hours of sleep should facilitate maximum productivity.

My particular six-hour pattern is not just about sleep. Other things are happening. My sleep is a physical, mental, emotional, and spiritual recovery process. I take inventory of my mental acuity throughout the day, because my actions are predicated on making clear decisions. In my case, six hours of quality sleep is much better than eight hours of restlessness.

If you're a person who believes they need ten to twelve hours, it's time to wake up! Do you know how many months you can add to your life with just six hours instead of twelve? We've already established that "now" would be a good time to start pursuing your Perfect Day, right? That every waking minute you will be making decisions that align with your North Star to *take* what you deserve.

Consider this mind-blowing fact for a moment: if you

spend the next forty years sleeping twelve hours per night, you will have slept for a total of 7,300 days. If you spend the next forty years sleeping six hours per night, you will have slept for a total of 3,650 days. The difference is that you spend 3,650 days awake rather than asleep.

THAT'S *TEN YEARS* ADDED TO YOUR CONSCIOUS LIFE.

I bet you'll think twice about sleeping in for longer than six hours now! There is no limit to what can be done with an extra two to four hours per day!

PRINCIPLE #1: YOUR BEDROOM IS YOUR SANCTUARY

To make the most of renewed energy, balancing rejuvenation vs. time spent sleeping is very important. It's not just about the hours of sleep—it's about the quality. One critical component of great sleep is a lack of light. If an element of light in the room interrupts complete darkness, studies show it prevents us from falling into the deep REM sleep we need for full rejuvenation. REM sleep is essential for the recovery process, so it's important to create an environment for it. Place blackout shades over your bedroom windows, turn off all electronics, and see how amazing sleep can really be!

PRINCIPLE #2: PRE-BED VISUALIZATION PROCESS

We've established that where your focus goes, your attention flows. The majority of us will wake up with a daily mission. For many of us, it's work or our business, and for others, it's parenting or schooling. Regardless of what your mission is, I've found it highly effective to deploy the following evening strategy to maximize your productivity.

Each night before bed, I'll write down everything I want to accomplish the next day. With certainty, I visualize myself completing each one of the tasks and vividly imagine how I will feel when it's accomplished. What sense of gratitude will I feel? How will this create happiness or health in my life? What sense of pride, confidence, and steadfastness will I feel once this list is conquered? I will then focus on these positive feelings for just five minutes before I crawl into my dark room and close my eyes.

There are nights when I don't practice this for various reasons, and there is a huge difference in my productivity the next day. By writing down everything you want to accomplish and creating mental and emotional certainty that it's done, you will wake up the following day in attack mode.

This is a prime example of living with purpose. I take this routine very seriously, and it's largely the reason I've been able to take Burn Boot Camp from a parking lot to a $100 million organization in just a few short years.

PRINCIPLE #3: NO LIGHTS, NO CAMERA, NO ACTION

In our home, Morgan and I have made the bedroom a sanctuary—it's designated for sleep and recovery. There's no TV in there, and we charge our phones in a different room. There's no LED glow from electronics, no random chirp from a text message or buzz if someone calls late at night. We don't allow the bedroom to be a place to conduct business or watch TV or movies. The living room is designated for entertainment and the office for business. For many years, we fell asleep with the TV on, and I noticed that even if I slept eight hours, the faint noise in the background never allowed me to reach the deep REM sleep required for rejuvenation. The "do not disturb" function on my iPhone has practically saved my life!

PRINCIPLE #4: KEEP IT COOL

Don't overlook your sleep environment. Temperature is another key element of a great night's sleep. While people sleep well at different temperatures, it's common to sleep soundly when the room is cooler. In my case, I'm hot-blooded with a very active metabolism, so I need to cool my body down in order to sleep well. I use a cold pad set at about fifty-five degrees that allows me to get comfortable, turn down my energy, and sleep well. Cold pads are available just about anywhere, and they're great when you share a bed with someone who wants layers of blankets and the temperature set at seventy-five degrees.

PRINCIPLE #5: GOOD NIGHT TEA

Now that we have darkness and temperature dialed in, let's talk about a nighttime rejuvenation drink. This is Tim Ferris's creation, and it is an easy-to-make elixir that helps me get quality sleep. It consists of six ounces of hot water, one freshly squeezed slice of lemon, one teaspoon of honey, and two tablespoons of apple cider vinegar. Stir it up, and drink it right before bed. There is no science behind why this drink is effective, other than my own personal experience and the claims of thousands of my successful clients. It helps relax your mind and drift into sound sleep.

My hope is that these strategies are effective suggestions to help rejuvenate your mind and body, bring more vitality to your day, and help you become happier and more self-aware. Experiment with these rituals until you find what works for you!

★ **CHAPTER 11** ★

THE PRINCIPLES OF SPIRITUAL MASTERY

This is not a book about religion. However, I will tell you that I'm a Christian. You don't have to believe in God, and I'm not upset with you if you don't. But chances are you believe in a higher power or a universal energy. Your spirituality is simply a connection between yourself and the universe.

For the purpose of coaching you in this chapter, I'll call it *faith*.

PRINCIPLE #1: DESIGN YOUR LIFE WITH FAITH

Wouldn't it be nice to already have all of your goals and dreams accomplished today? Wouldn't it be a wise thing for you to do if you had the ability? Good news: that ability lives in every one of us!

Faith is simply knowing that something exists, even if it isn't physically there.

When I started Burn Boot Camp, I saw a giant metaphorical skyscraper when everyone else around me saw a vacant piece of land. We all have the ability to accomplish goals inside of ourselves before they ever physically manifest. This ability is in our DNA as human beings.

Think about your Perfect Day. It may not be here physically for years, but you have the opportunity to spiritually, mentally, and emotionally *finish it* right now. This book has given you a whole new psychology, as I've provided you with new ways to think, shift your paradigm, and overcome your former excuses. I've introduced you to actuality and kicked your former reality to the curb.

THE TRUTH IS, YOU'LL BE SOMEWHERE IN FIVE YEARS. THE QUESTION IS, *WHERE* WILL YOU BE?

Will you choose to be stuck in the same place, or will you choose to deploy the lessons of this book to manifest lasting change in your life?

You're going to be someplace else in five years, and the question is, *where will you be?* In a worse place, the same place, or a better place? I know where you don't want to be: a place you didn't design for yourself. This is where you'll end up if you wait for someone else's permission, fail to redefine yourself, and never question why you think the way you do. You have the gift of choice, so use it to design your own life!

I challenge you to walk through the valley of the shadow of death. Why? Not because I want you to like demons, but because there is light at the end of the valley. It's time to start living life as if it's rigged in your favor.

So often we go through life feeling like victims, but there is no such thing. There are only volunteers. You've chosen the life you've lived, and you will choose what the future holds for you tomorrow.

Even the worst heartbreak is part of the process, and how you use the event determines its ultimate meaning. When you truly believe that life happens *for* you and not *to* you, all of the frustration, overwhelm, and stress is viewed as a gift from the universe.

Faith is *knowing* with conviction that all of the universe is compounding over time to create your experience of life. That is faith. When your focus lies on the world being against you, you'll suffer great pain. When you wake up in a beautiful state of being and believe that life is rigged in your favor, you will open up the opportunity to experience Grace.

Have faith that when you take the actions that align with your North Star on a consistent basis, you will inevitably reach your long-term goals. It won't always be today or tomorrow, and usually, you'll take an unforeseen path to get there, but you *will* get there. It won't be today and doesn't have to be tomorrow, but when you're certain about something, it eventually shows up in your life.

Faith will bring about joy in your life's day-to-day operations, and you won't always be searching to achieve your expectations. I urge you to have a big vision and believe in the power of what your Perfect Day will bring you.

When you think this way, you open up your world to a whole lot of opportunity to receive Grace from the universe. Success in anything takes intentional activity, hustling your ass off, and a relentless belief that you will accomplish your goals. There is no such thing as luck. Luck is simply the point in time when preparation meets opportunity.

PRINCIPLE #2: CONNECTING TO THE UNIVERSE

I'm going to teach you a spiritual ritual that I've incorporated into my life that allows me to connect to the universe on a daily basis. My teacher, Tony Robbins, taught me this practice, and I thought it was stupid at first. I was reluctant to use it, and thought it was psychotherapy bullshit.

I finally decided to do it one morning as I felt a lack of connection with the universe, and it was such a powerful experience that I've done it nearly every day since.

For this to work, you must play this all out. There's no getting around the fact that you may be turned off by this at first. This may sound a little corny and esoteric, but we all know the definition of insanity by now, right? You will need some Grace along the path to reaching your fitness goals, and this practice will allow you receive Grace with open arms.

1. You must be in solitude when you do this exercise. It can be done at any time of the day.
2. Close your eyes and breathe in and out through your nose very rapidly for thirty seconds. At the end of thirty seconds, with your eyes closed, think of one thing you are particularly grateful for. Focus on how this makes you feel. Repeat three times.
3. Upon conclusion of your third set, raise both hands to the sky as high as you can. Vividly imagine yourself grabbing ahold of the universal energy you believe in. (I usually envision a blue light of energy swirling around my hands.)
4. Envision pulling this energy to your body with your hands. Place them on your head for a moment, and give the energy to *your* brain as you massage your skull. Let the energy then circulate in your heart for

a few moments, and feel your heart beating. Lastly, imagine the energy shooting down your legs and out the bottom of your feet into the earth.

5. Imagine the energy travels down to the earth's core and collects even more intensity. The energy then shoots back up into your body through your legs and into your heart with more intensity than before. Imagine sharing this energy with your coworkers, family, and friends by shooting the blue energy from your palms to their hearts.

6. Lastly, repeat this practice five times with the energy, body movements, and visualizations that dramatically intensify with each repetition.

The feeling after you commit yourself 100 percent to this exercise for the first time will get you hooked. The universe is real, and its power is abundant. I challenge you practice this every day for ten straight days. If you want to magnetically attract what you ultimately desire in your life, I highly recommend doing this.

If you're still thinking that this is nonsense, since when did you become so grown-up? What's wrong with being playful and fun? There's nothing to lose here, and everything to gain. The power you will attract in your life from practicing this consistently cannot be put into words.

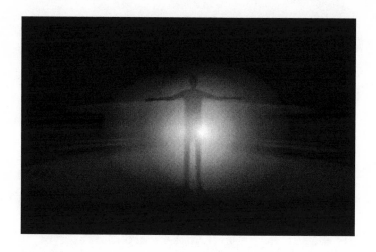

PRINCIPLE #3: THE LAW OF REAPING AND SOWING

There are universal laws that will always affect you no matter what stage of life you're in. Some of them are physical, but others are quantum (spiritual). There are dozens of spiritual laws, but I am going to teach you one universal law that will impact your life right now!

By human nature, we tend to gravitate to complicated strategies and generally disregard the simple ones. It's the simple ideas in life that have the greatest impact. We hear them so often that they become white noise and seem clichéd, when in reality, they are laws of the universe that are absolute. Complexity is the enemy of all execution, and simplicity is the friend of success.

I'm going to teach you the very simple universal law of

reaping and sowing. This law says that whatever you plant in your mind, you will manifest in your physical reality—that whatever you think about most often, you will become.

Your mind is just like a garden, and you get to choose the seeds that are planted. Planting an apple seed will manifest into an apple tree with sunlight, water, and soil. As humans, our goals are the seeds, your brain is the soil, your thoughts are the water, and your feelings are the sun. When you expose yourself to this type of nurturing, the seeds must become flowers. Planting a seed and not reinforcing it with nutrients and environmental elements will stunt the growth of the seed, and it will die.

THE PROBLEM IS THAT MOST HUMAN BEINGS THINK ABOUT WHAT THEY *DON'T WANT* TO ATTRACT, RATHER THAN WHAT THEY *DO WANT* TO ATTRACT.

We have this list of goals we want to accomplish, but without reinforcing them on a daily basis with our rituals, we forget to revisit the goals, and our dreams dissolve in our brains. Instead, we spend our spiritual and mental energy thinking about the things we don't want. "I don't want to be overweight anymore," "I don't want to be broke anymore," and "I don't want to feel run down anymore." Remember those six words I asked you to remember at the very beginning of this book? *Whatever you think about you will become.*

Conscious observers of life create their own actuality. I'm telling you this because this has transformed my life in so many ways. When I realized that my life was a garden and I got to choose which seeds I planted, how often I watered them, and how much sun exposure I would give them, my life started to explode.

Even if you do understand, this is where you're most likely lacking patience. There are seasons of reaping and sowing. In some seasons of life, you eat the fruit that you've harvested all summer. In other seasons, the pests come along and eat all your fruit, and in others, you won't get any rain. But what you always have to realize is that you will eventually reap what you sow. Whether positive or negative, the vibe you put out will come back to you.

It's your decision whether or not you plant fruit trees or allow weeds to grow, but the law of reaping and sowing will always be a universal principle that exists in our world.

You have to realize that your mind is a garden, and weeds will grow without your permission. I'm not telling you to stand outside of your garden and chant, "There are no weeds; there are no weeds; there are no weeds." I suggest you dig your hand into the dirt and rip them out by their roots. They are your negative thoughts, and they will make their way into your head if you allow them.

Your thoughts will always precede your actions. Imagine what it will feel like when you accomplish your goals. Think about what your life will be like one, five, and ten years from now when you plant seeds of positivity today. What freedom will you have? How will this affect your children?

Plant seeds of hard work, gratitude, love, understanding, and unrelenting desire to wake up and attack your goals every day. Life is a constant cycle of reaping and sowing. Whatever energy you put into the universe, you will get back. What you focus on, you will feel. This is a simple law, and when you master the simple practicality of this, you can attract anything you want into your life.

★ CHAPTER 12 ★

OVERCOMING OBJECTIONS

OBJECTION #1: I'VE TRIED "EVERYTHING"

The first and most common objection I hear from new clients is "I've tried everything." This is transformative language at its finest, and when people tell me this, my investigative curiosity kicks in.

My response is always "Okay, so you've tried everything? A Google search yields about 420 *million* nutrition strategies, so it should be no problem for you to list one hundred, right? List one hundred of those strategies you've tried."

No one has ever been able to give me one hundred strategies. They usually respond with "That's a hard one. I've just tried so many different things, and nothing seems to work."

Next, I lower the number and ask them to list ten strategies. Typically, a client will say something like, "Okay, I've been on and off with Weight Watchers, I've done the Atkins Diet a few times, and most recently, I tried Whole30."

"Okay, so that's three strategies. Can you give me seven more?"

"I guess I those are the only things I've tried."

"So, have you *really* tried everything? It sounds like you've tried the same three strategies over and over with similar results. Would you say this is true?"

At that point in the conversation, the client realizes they haven't tried everything—they've tried the same two or three things over and over with no results, or similar results each time. That is the definition of insanity: attempting the same actions or events repeatedly, and expecting different results. You aren't an insane person, but when you say you've tried everything, the truth is you've tried the same few things repeatedly. It's time to get rid of this objection. You haven't tried everything, because if you had, you wouldn't still be looking for a strategy that works. It's time to change your approach.

Are you up for the challenge of trying something new? My main goal in this section is to encourage you to open yourself up to options! Most of us go on a "diet," restrict calories, and deprive ourselves of the foods we enjoy.

I'm here to tell you that you can eat processed food and binge on sugar, but you can also eat healthy foods that create energy and vitality in your life. You have every option available to you, and you're 100 percent in control of which ones you choose.

There's more than one way to reach your goals, and I promise that if you continue to follow your North Star and don't make U-turns, you will get there. If a particular approach doesn't work, we'll change it. If that new strategy doesn't work, we'll change it again. We'll continue to change the approach until we find the strategy that works for you. As long as you're open to trying new things and never give up, you'll eventually find what works for you.

Can we agree that you haven't tried "everything"? If you want to achieve something new, you must *do* something new. This applies to all areas of your life, not just your fitness goals.

YOU WOULDN'T TREAT YOUR CHILDREN THIS WAY

I remember when my daughter Cameron turned one

and attempted to walk for the first time. She stood up on wobbly legs, swayed side to side, tried to take a step, and fell on her butt. Not once did I think, "Well, I guess my daughter just isn't a walker." That would have been ridiculous, right? Instead of giving up, we tried a new approach. I placed a chair in front of her and made her stand up holding the chair. She fell over. Then, I held her hands to assist her until her knees gave out. When that didn't work, we went back to the drawing board. No parent in this situation would say, "I've tried everything, and nothing works for her." You'd keep trying until your child was able to do sprints around the coffee table. There's no other choice! This is *exactly* how we need to treat our fitness goals.

There must be a point when you realize one strategy isn't working, and you say, "I'm not giving up. This is what I'm achieving, no matter how long it takes." You haven't tried everything until you're successful and thriving. Once you've established this strong foundational mindset of absolute certainty, you'll never start over again. Constant and consistent progression will create happiness in your life.

LAG VS. LEAD MEASUREMENTS

Hope is an awful strategy. Saying, "I hope I reach my goals," is like saying, "I'll just close my eyes, and the results might magically appear." If you want to reach your goals, you need to understand the difference between *lag* and *lead measurements*. You cannot manage what you don't measure. The following tip will delete hope from the brain and install certainty that you'll reach your desired outcome.

A lag measurement is long-term and *is* the outcome—it shows whether or not you are close to achieving your goal. Lead measurements are short-term drivers that "lead" to your specific outcome. For example, if your desired outcome is to lose twelve pounds in three months, that's a lag measurement. The lead measurements are the caloric deficit, frequency of workout sessions, and quantity of water you drink daily to make sure the lag measurement is achieved.

Hoping and praying to step on the scale in three months and see that it reads twelve pounds lighter will leave you disappointed. It takes a caloric deficit of 3,500 calories to lose one pound. If you want to lose twelve pounds in twelve weeks, you need to create a daily deficit of 500 calories. Measuring your caloric intake and creating a daily deficit of 500 calories is an intermediate measurement—it helps you to be absolutely sure you'll reach the lag measurement. By using this strategy, you'll never have to "hope" again, and you will be certain to achieve your goals.

OBJECTION #2: NOT ENOUGH ENERGY

Through the past six years of case studies and working with many people, a common objection to getting started on the path to health is a lack of energy. People say, "I just can't spend energy on this because it drains me for the rest of the day," or, "I don't have enough energy at the end of the day to head to the gym."

Let's be brutally honest for a moment. This is a ridiculous thought pattern! That's like saying, "I want to make money, but I don't want to work." The only way to get energy is to ignite physiology, and the best way to ignite physiology is through movement of the body. If you want more energy but say you don't have enough, it's no different than wanting to lose weight and then eating an entire pie for dessert every night. Step outside your reality, employ your actuality, and become aware of what you are saying.

We have two abundant resources inside of us that require zero talent or unique skill: energy and hustle. Sometimes, we just have to dig down and pull them out, and reading your North Star statement aloud helps you do this. A key ingredient to long-term transformation is *perseverance*. I define perseverance as working hard after you've already worked hard.

If you physically don't have enough energy, take a look at your diet, and be honest. How many times have you eaten processed food this week? How much water have you consumed today? By intuition alone, would you say your body is alkaline or acidic? Having energy is a choice. If you've ever felt like skipping a workout but then decided to do it anyway, you know how much better you feel afterwards. Projection is a powerful tool, and if you put yourself in the state of being after a workout, it paints a picture of how you know you will feel. You just have to make the choice to do it!

Your goals don't care about your feelings. If you really want your fitness to change, *you* have to change. If you want life to get better, *you* have to get better. You may not like me for saying this, but it's true. It's time to stop telling yourself bullshit stories that paint you as the victim and your circumstances as the villain. When your priorities align with your North Star, you'll never use the excuse of not having energy again, because you'll have a reason to work out that is stronger than any feelings of lack you may experience.

I BET YOU'D HAVE ENERGY FOR THIS

If I offered you $5 million to meet me at the beach at 4:30 a.m. and run sprints for an hour every morning for one week, would you do it? Show me anyone who says "no" to this offer, and I'll show you a liar. So, when you say you don't have enough energy, what you're *really* saying is it's not important; there's no motivator pulling you toward it. Change is not a matter of ability but rather a matter of motivation.

In this scenario, think of the $5 million as your North

Star—the money pulls you toward the goal. Thinking about all you could do with this money gives you strong motivation. The reason for showing up is so compelling that you don't even question getting up when that alarm goes off. You're so excited that you can barely sleep! There's nothing that stops you from being on that beach. Heck, you'd probably show up early, get a warm-up in, and do it with a smile on your face!

Now, let this blow your mind. You'd do this for $5 million, but money isn't nearly as important as your health, vitality, family, and happiness, is it? Doesn't your health and happiness give you a higher quality of life than money ever could? I have dozens of CEO friends who are rich and miserable. What more motivation do you need? It's time to get your priorities aligned with what truly matters.

BURN YOUR BOATS

In order to create lasting change, you must eliminate the stories that create limiting beliefs. You must exhaust all options other than achieving what success means to you, or in other words, your Perfect Day. Have you ever heard the phrase "To take over the islands, you must burn your boats"? This popular analogy is used by many motivational speakers, but what does it mean?

Imagine your goal is to take over an island, but enemy soldiers are defending the borders. As you approach the island and park the boats ashore, you become fearful of what may happen. As your men begin to storm the island, the general yells out, "Burn the boats!" Your soldiers ask the general why he would do such a thing. The general replies, "When you burn the boats, we only have two options: take the island, or die trying."

If the general hadn't ordered for the boats to be set on fire, then your men would have been equipped for another option: to turn around and sail back home, thus not reaching their goal of taking over the island. By burning the boats, the general fully committed his troops to accomplishing their goal.

The "boats" in your life are the excuses you've used in the past to quit and start over later. The "islands" in your life are the goals you've been attacking for years. If you want to take the islands, burn the boats and leave yourself with no option other than goal achievement. The answer to the question "How do I stop starting over and create lasting change?" is simpler than it's ever been: burn your boats.

To paraphrase a famous quote by Will Smith, if you and I get on a treadmill together, one of two things will happen: either you get off, or I die on the treadmill." This is the type of mentality you need to dominate any goal in your life. The strategy to implement this mentality is simple: make the choice to create the resolve. We have the ability to make a life-changing choice at any time, and I believe that is one of the greatest and most underused powers of human beings.

OBJECTION #3: TIME VS. PRIORITIES

It's a classic story. "I don't have time to exercise."

I have a hunch that you've heard someone utter this phrase before. This is by far the most common objection I hear. Rather than saying, "I don't have enough energy," it's easier to say, "I don't have time," because you get to point the blame at everything that consumes it.

I'll come right out and say it: it's *never* that you don't have the time. It's *always* that you haven't made yourself a priority yet. So many of us allow our perception of time to control our behaviors. We live with the idea that we serve time, and it does not serve us. "There's only so much time in the day" is a poor excuse—it all comes down to how you prioritize your time. We all have the same opportunity with the same twenty-four hours. In actuality, you've got the time to achieve everything you desire and more. You need to take control of time and "command" it to work for you.

We know that when you ask better questions, you'll get better answers. "How do I work out when I don't have the time?" is a poor question. You're assuming that time controls your life. Ask yourself a better question, like, "When can I make the time to work out?" This question assumes that you have the time; you simply have to leverage it appropriately. I never ask myself, "Why aren't there more hours in the day?" but rather "How much can I accomplish in every hour of every day?"

Believing you don't have enough time is another way of saying your goal isn't important enough for you—it's not your priority. Do you realize that everything you want to manifest in your life starts and stops with the strength of your psychology? When you are your number one priority, you'll make the time to be healthy and happy by default. Get up thirty minutes earlier or go to bed later. Trade your ninety minutes of Facebook or your binge on Netflix for productive activities that create a maximized quality of life. You always have the time, and I'll prove it to you, if you're willing to take the following exercise seriously.

168 HOURS: WHAT WILL YOU DO WITH THEM?

Right now, we're going to walk through an exercise that I've made a routine part of my life. Putting this into practice allowed me to clearly realize that lack of time is an illusion. My mindset shifted from "I only have an hour—

that's not enough time" to "I have an hour—how much can I get done?" I do this exercise every January to make sure I'm not wasting a moment of my time. In fact, the first time I did this exercise, I discovered forty hours each week that I could use more efficiently. This exercise puts the actuality of how much time is available in front of your face, so if you're serious about changing, I highly suggest you complete this exercise.

168-Hour Time-Bucket Exercise

To begin this exercise, take out your cell phone, open your notes, and write "Time Buckets" and the date at the top. Knowing there are 168 hours in every week, you'll take inventory of every hour and place them in different categories, or buckets. This exercise requires a one-week commitment—you'll record how much time you spend on each of your activities in a normal week.

Every day for seven days, "clock in" and "clock out" of everything you do. Take a committed inventory of every hour of time: eating lunch, writing emails, talking on the phone, spending time with your kids, sleeping, working, etc. This can be tedious, but it's temporary, and it will be worth it. You can have an "ah-ha" moment similar to mine with this time-bucket exercise!

The Buckets

Record how much time you spend on each of the following categories, or buckets:

★ **Mission Bucket:** This is your job, career, school, community involvement, volunteer work, etc.—anything you do to create financial freedom or to give back to your community.

★ **Family Bucket:** These are the *dedicated* hours you spend with them. Sitting in the living room working on your laptop doesn't count; that's work. This is playing with your kids, conversing with your spouse, or spending time with family members.

★ **Leisure Bucket:** This includes socializing with friends, going out to dinner, sporting events, or anything else you do for fun with your friends.

★ **Eating Bucket:** Record the time you spend eating/meal prepping and doing nothing else.

★ **Screen Bucket:** This includes social media (not for work), TV, Netflix, or any other time you stare at a screen for pleasure.

★ **Sleep Bucket:** Record the time you go to bed and the time you wake up.

★ **"Me" Bucket:** This is time spent exercising, reading, or working on personal development—anything you do to better yourself.

I've done the time-bucket exercise with a large majority of

my 20,000 clients, and the results have been staggering. On average, we uncovered about forty hours per week of unproductive leisure activities, like binge-watching Netflix, mindlessly scrolling through Facebook, staring at sports events on TV, and other unproductive actions that focused on *other* people's lives. Much of this wasted time was spent watching others, like friends and professional athletes, be successful. If you're watching others chase their dreams, then yours are running farther away from you! Imagine what you could do with another forty hours per week dedicated to your North Star!

If your Perfect Day is to work an eight-to-five job, play on every softball or volleyball team, and go drinking with friends on the weekends, go forth and be happy. Everyone's definition of success is different, and I'm not suggesting you live anyone else's life. This book is about designing *your* life and creating lasting change on *your* terms. If your happiness aligns with spending lots of time doing leisure activities, that's great! Just don't complain when your situation doesn't improve. If you make the choice to spend forty hours a week doing things that don't progress your mission, your family, or losing weight, don't bitch and moan when you are stuck in the same place.

The time-bucket exercise uncovers how many hours you spend doing things that don't align with your North Star, giving you the opportunity to make choices and reallocate your time. Any hour that is not spent in alignment should be considered wasted time, and you need to make adjustments—begin incorporating rituals that will bring you closer to your goals.

I've found that tapping into about 20 percent of wasted time is all it takes to expand your opportunities and reach the next level in your career, health, or family life—to get closer to your Perfect Day. The time-bucket exercise provides you with facts, and there's no arguing with them— the information will be right in front of you, confirming where you spend your time.

This exercise gives you the opportunity to design your life and deploy all of the mental, emotional, physical, and spiritual rituals suggested to stop starting over. If you want results, you have to take action. Your lifestyle has to lead without internal conflict. If you want to make more money, then turn off Netflix and work on your side hustle. If you want to lose weight and think you've tried everything, think of what you do from 6:00 to 10:00 p.m. every night. Instead of watching reality TV, go for an hour-long run. You can watch TV later. Reduce the time you spend on activities that don't align with your outcomes.

It doesn't matter if you have five kids, two jobs, and a needy spouse. It doesn't matter if the dog peed on the floor and the baby is screaming. You *always* have the ability to free up at least an hour for yourself! I've coached my clients through this exercise for the past several years, and the majority of them have taken action. Align your time with your goals, and you move one step closer to achieving them. The harsh actuality is, if you don't have an hour per day to focus on your own happiness, you don't have a life.

OBJECTION #4: I'M NOT A FITNESS PERSON

This is a perfect example of transformational language patterns. Once clients enter the Burn Boot Camp program, our expert certified personal trainers take them through a series of one-on-one Focus Meetings. Everything I'm teaching you in this book is derived from the successful outcomes of these meetings, with real people just like you. Focus Meetings uncover gaps in their psychology, and we discuss everything you are reading in this book over a long period of time. A common objection I encounter as an excuse for not committing to their journey is "I'm just not a fitness person."

What must first be recognized about this objection is the language—it's transformative! Do you see how transformative language can be extremely poisonous to the mind? If you say you're "not a fitness person," you corner yourself into that limiting belief system. Through past experiences or preconditioning, you adopted a language pattern that solidifies this false statement, and it traps you in mediocrity. Since you have this identity, you'll do whatever is necessary to maintain that identity. As human beings, we always behave in accordance with who we believe we are. You might not say, "I'm not a fitness person," but you might say, "I could never do a pull-up." Or, "I'm just not strong enough." If you truly believe you could never do a pull-up, why would you even practice?

Once you are comfortable with an identity, it tends to stick with you, regardless of any outside, positive influences. If you believe you're not a fitness person, your focus will find everything in life that aligns with that belief. How silly does it sound to define yourself as "not a fitness person"? No one is born doing burpees out of the womb. The doctor doesn't say, "Congratulations! You have a fitness baby!" You picked up a belief along the way that subconsciously created this identity. By human nature, you'll do *everything* possible to stay consistent with the belief of who you are, even when a greater quality of life is knocking at your door.

Have I quashed your objection yet? I want to be real with you. This is a book of practical psychology—let's call it "practichology"—and there are ways to interrupt your habitual, unproductive thought processes and replace them with new ones. Can you spread your feet shoulder width apart right now and drop down to do one body squat? Can you do one jumping jack? One push-up on your knees? Lift five pounds over your head? If you answered "yes" to any of those, we've just confirmed that you *are*, in fact, capable of being a person who practices fitness!

You are capable of practicing fitness every single day, even if you only do two squats tomorrow and three the next day. It's never that you can't do it; it's that you haven't done it *yet!* Don't be the elephant that can't tear the stake out of the ground and run free because she believes "it is what it is."

OBJECTION #5: MONEY IS A PROBLEM

The second most-common objection I hear—and one that most everyone says at some point—is "I don't have enough money to get fit." I want you to get up right now, drop to your knees, and do five push-ups. Seriously, give it a shot. How much money did that cost? Need I say more?

Does the definition of getting fit say you need to spend money? It doesn't, and if you think it does, it's time to get rid of that notion. You pay taxes, and the roads are yours to run! Ask a trainer how to get fit for free, and she will tell you there are millions of strategies out there. I'm a practical person, and $150-a-month gym memberships can simply be too far out of reach, especially for someone working two jobs to support four kids. As mentioned in the previous chapter, you can do bodyweight exercises at home for free, or join Morgan and me on YouTube.

"But I'm one hundred pounds overweight, and I've never exercised in my life." Then don't run—go for a walk. Do *anything* to move your body. If you think you've already tried a bunch of strategies, try another one!

I post weekly videos on Instagram. All you have to do is watch and participate. My YouTube channel is also free. Follow along and get fit. Don't have internet at home? Go to a library or coffee shop, watch the videos, and then head to the parking lot to work out. Be resourceful!

You could also save a few bucks by giving up some small luxuries here and there. I follow the "coffee rule." The average Frappuccino or latte at your local java house is five or six dollars. If that's your fix, trade the six bucks and extra calories for a gym membership, new running shoes, or something that will help you reach your North Star. Maybe you're not a coffee drinker, but you like smoothies, frequent the taco buffet at a local pub, or get breakfast from a bagel shop every morning. Any one of those can cost up to eight bucks per day. Ditching them will create energy, better health, and financial freedom to join a gym if you're not intrinsically motivated.

If you're not a coffee nut and still want to be smart with your money, you can hack your grocery bill. Buying organic foods in bulk from places like Costco and Walmart is surprisingly affordable. Storing food in the freezer allows you to keep healthy foods on hand, and you can reallocate grocery funds toward a gym membership or fitness gear.

Look around and figure out what luxuries or habits you could eliminate. If you think about what's really happening, it's another version of your reality that needs to be questioned. All the objections—I don't have time, I don't have enough money, I'm not a fitness person, and I don't have enough energy—are ways of saying fitness is not a priority. When you burn your boats, the decision to take over the island is easy.

★ CHAPTER 13 ★

THE MAGIC OF MOMENTUM

Now, we are going to take everything we've discussed and bring it together. Don't be overwhelmed—I've crammed several years of my findings into this book. Don't expect to wake up tomorrow and use every strategy. I want you to realize that taking action on even one of my mental, emotional, physical, or spiritual principles can begin to create lasting change in your life. This is a process, and you must trust, enjoy, and own it.

Before we dive into a powerful concept that I call the "Magic of Momentum," I'd like to offer you some encouragement. I want you to think about our privilege as human beings. When a dog stares at the night sky, it's often said that it is "looking to the moon." When a dog looks at the moon, it sees a light. Period. There are no thoughts about what the moon is, why it's there, how it got there, or why it's part of the universe. The same is true for all other creatures on earth, aside from humans—they don't question existence. Humans have the gift of wonder. We can ponder how snow is created before it falls from the sky, why the wind blows, or the physics behind sending a person to the moon. We should be grateful for our ability to ask these questions, and use it to advance in our journey to health.

Our brains allow us to have unique, individual mindsets capable of tremendous thought. We can decide who we want to be tomorrow, and we can question what happened for us yesterday. It's a wonderful gift, knowing you're in complete control. As long as you place 90 percent of your focus on your psychology and 10 percent on the strategy, you'll be standing on a platform to begin what I call the Magic of Momentum.

I believe it is our responsibility as human beings to question who we are and what our purpose is, and to take full advantage of endless possibilities to create a better life. When you use the Magic of Momentum appropriately, life's possibilities transform into *probabilities*, and understanding this one concept will put everything we've talked about into perspective.

THE MAGIC OF MOMENTUM CYCLE

To create momentum in our lives, we must continually take incremental steps to reach our goals. I call this the "Magic of Momentum Cycle." This cycle has four parts:

1. **Belief**—the thoughts we have about achievement
2. **Action**—what we do about those thoughts
3. **Results**—what we achieve from the action
4. **Potential**—the reinforcement of belief

The Magic of Momentum Cycle starts with a belief about what's possible for our lives. The level of belief you have determines the actions you take. The actions you take will determine the results you experience. The results you experience are given a meaning. The meaning you give to an experience will determine the future potential of your beliefs.

When you've burned your boats and there's no way you're *not* reaching your goal, you've got maximum belief. Come hell or high water, you'll do whatever it takes to get there. If you have a whatever-it-takes mentality and a committed belief, you'll take committed action. You might even take massive action! If you take massive action, what kind of results will you get? Massive results! Once you get those results, the potential of your abilities increases—you boost the belief in yourself. When your potential boosts your belief, you'll take *even more action* yielding *even better results*. This is the Magic of Momentum Cycle!

MAGIC OF MOMENTUM

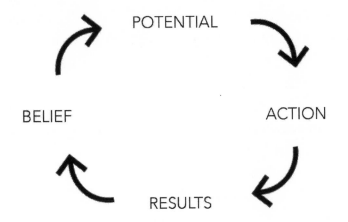

POTENTIAL

BELIEF

ACTION

RESULTS

THE BRANDI PARKER STORY

I want to share a story with you to about a client named Brandi Parker. Brandi's story brings to light the Magic of Momentum and how this can be a powerful realization for you.

I distinctly remember the day when I met Brandi, because there was so much emotion attached to it, and it helped define me as a trainer. I had a 5:30 a.m. session with about thirty regular clients. I was hyped and motivated, the music was cranked, and the atmosphere was killer.

My training session had already started this day, and it was like God tapped me on the shoulder. He turned my attention away from training clients and toward the doorway of the gym. As I felt this vibe, I looked toward the lobby and noticed an obese woman had stepped into the room. I immediately sensed she was fearful, and I felt an "Oh shoot, he saw me" energy coming from her.

A voice in my head said, "Go help this woman," and without hesitation, I sprinted over to the door. She didn't see me at first, and I said, "Hey, hold on! Hi, how are you? My name is Devan. Nice to meet you. What's your name?"

She was very shy. Her shoulders were slouched, and her eyes were glued to the floor. "Hi," she replied timidly. "I'm Brandi Parker."

I'm sure I was an intimidating presence to a woman who was tipping the scale at almost 400 pounds. My physical appearance and energy overwhelmed her, so I decided to slide around next to her and place my arm around her shoulders. I wanted to comfort her and make her feel as if we were already buddies.

She continued to look down, and I sternly said, "Hey, can you look at me for a second?" When she looked up, I said, "You belong here, Brandi." She smiled from ear to ear. This small moment planted the seed of belief that Brandi needed. I could tell she didn't believe in herself, so I knew I had to get the cycle of momentum started immediately.

No one had ever believed in Brandi before, and by planting the seed of belief, I persuaded her to stay and perform the next step in the cycle: action. Brandi had a hard time getting out of the car and walking in the door, let alone doing one of my crazy Burn Boot Camp sessions, but she agreed to come and work out. I connected with her through the next thirty minutes, intentionally installing more belief with every movement and repetition.

I didn't bring her to the front of the gym and put her on display. I ran the session with a mic on, but I trained Brandi one-on-one, as she had confined herself to a two-by-two corner in the back of the gym. Instead of doing traditional push-ups on the floor, Brandi and I did them against the wall. Instead of doing jump squats, we did standing, low-impact high knees; and instead of jumping rope, she chopped her feet over and back on the edge of my raised gymnastics floor.

We did exercises she could handle, and it helped her feel like she fit in—she felt good about the action she was taking. She gave 100 percent that day, and I let her know that it was not only good enough—it was amazing! Understanding the next step in the cycle, I asked her questions so she would intentionally feel the results of her newfound belief and decision to take action.

"What you're doing today is incredible. How do you feel

about today? How do you feel about going through this workout?" I asked her.

She answered with a smile. "Well, I feel much better than when I started. I didn't think I could do it, but I guess I was wrong!" And just like that, she got her first taste of results, after the very first workout.

"Are you still standing?" I asked jokingly. She answered "yes," and I asked her how she felt.

"I feel better. I feel empowered. I even feel a little more confident already." She stacked more results on her subconscious record.

"Not only did you do it, you crushed it! I expect you to show up tomorrow!" I jokingly demanded this, knowing that I needed to get her buy-in. Once she took the action of doing a camp and felt the results, the last step was to reinforce that she could feel even better if she came back. By asking, "Are you coming back?" I really meant, "Do you believe you can do this again?"

"Yes, I'm going to come back," she replied confidently.

As a means to further reinforce her belief in herself, I let her know she wasn't alone. "If you give me the chance to show you that this is different from every other strategy you've tried, I promise I can help change your life. I'll be your friend and walk with you every step of the way." We exchanged numbers, and later, I texted her encouraging words. Sure enough, it worked, and she showed up again.

She came back day after day at 5:30 a.m. Each time we had camp, we went through another Magic of Momentum Cycle as I intentionally installed more positive beliefs into Brandi. She began feeling better and began losing weight quickly. These beliefs led to Brandi's dedicated action, and she could hear, feel, and see the results before her own eyes. The other ladies in camp began to praise Brandi for the amazing job she was doing. Her repeated action of coming to camp and seeing results continued to reinforce her beliefs—that this could be the strategy that worked for her.

After two months of coming in five days per week, she saw significant results, and I was beginning to see a trans-formed person. The cycle was fully engaged. With a little dedication and effort, she not only accomplished something she never had before, she also gained the belief that she could keep going. During our Focus Meetings, we used my "projection of pain" method to ensure that she wouldn't take any steps backwards or become complacent.

INSPIRATION SPARKS A TRANSFORMATION

I'm partnered with Shaklee, the world's largest natural nutrition-supplement company and the creators of the multivitamin. Shortly after I met Brandi and she started crushing it, I attended our Shaklee Global Conference event in Las Vegas, and there was a speaker named Jacqui McCoy. She had lost several hundred pounds and was featured on Chris and Heidi Powell's *Extreme Weight Loss* television show—she was one of their most successful transformation stories. I've always looked up to Chris as an influence in my life in terms of his ability to motivate people to accomplish amazing weight loss feats. The unique thing about Chris is that all his clients, by their own estimation, are too far gone to ever take back control of their lives.

When I heard Jacqui pour out her heart on stage in front of 4,000 people, I was utterly moved. I had followed Chris and Jacqui's journey, and her speech made me see the parallels to Brandi and me. I immediately became certain that whether she liked it or not, we were going to kick this momentum cycle into high gear!

I ditched the rest of the conference, ran up to my hotel room, and spent three hours putting together a one-year transformation program for Brandi and me to embark on. I planned for her to come to Burn five days a week, with extra one-on-one workouts with me in the parking lot two evenings a week. I also designed a dedicated nutrition plan built around Shaklee's Life Supplement line. It consisted of meal replacement shakes, snack bars, and meal bars to give her turnkey options to lose weight healthily and quickly. I emailed the plan to her and told her I was committed, if she was willing to do it. She agreed. Brandi didn't realize it at the time, but all of her newfound belief led her to commit to taking massive action—like committing to a twelve-month plan that took three hours to create!

We implemented exercises and rituals to intentionally continue the cycle. I had a Dodge Challenger at the time, and I made her push the car down the street while I sat inside and feathered the brakes to add resistance. It was a blend of strength training and empowerment. I told her if she can push a car, she can lose the weight. Her belief was at an all-time high!

Within a year, the Magic of Momentum was proven. Brandi almost walked out of Burn on the first day, but one ounce of potential snowballed into mountains of belief! To think, Brandi almost never started because of fear and insecurity from her past, but one vote of confidence led to her losing an amazing 174 pounds. She created a completely new physical, mental, and emotional life. This powerful revolving momentum continues today!

Something she said at the end of training brought me

to tears. "It's so cool that now I can get on an airplane without having to ask for a seatbelt extender." I'll never forget that, because her statement gave me insight into the struggles of people who consume too much food and end up in circumstances they never intended. Brandi didn't just lose nearly 200 pounds; she also gained control over all areas of her life. It was the most gratifying feeling of my life, next to getting married and having children. Brandi's success reinforced my own belief in how great a trainer I could be, so I guess she did just as much for me as I did for her.

Since Brandi could now run to the mailbox and far beyond, I surprised her with a half-marathon trail run together at the end of her transformation program. It was a run through the woods, and we jumped over roots and dodged bushes. It was fantastic! As we crossed the finish line, we shared an emotional hug. I'll never forget that moment! Do you think Brandi thought she would be running a half-marathon in twelve months when she first walked into Burn? No way! The Magic of Momentum cycle is extremely powerful!

THE CYCLE WORKS BOTH WAYS

As awesome as Brandi's story is, you must be careful, because the Magic of Momentum can work the opposite way, too. If you don't believe that the teachings in this book will work for you, will you take a lot or a little action after you're done reading? A little. If you take a little action on my recommendations, will you get great results or poor results? Poor. If you get poor results, you'll only reinforce a negative belief, and you'll convince yourself that your original belief was correct. You'll find yourself saying, "I knew all of this stupid psychology stuff wouldn't work."

This can be a vicious cycle. Do yourself a favor, and use this book as your positive momentum. Use Brandi's story as inspiration to unleash your potential. She wasn't an athlete; she had been overweight her whole life and weighed nearly 400 pounds. She didn't have a unique talent or skill set, and she didn't find a magic potion. Brandi used one nugget of potential and redesigned her entire life, because she believed that taking consistent action would lead to results.

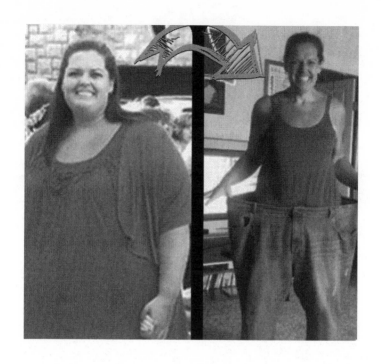

★ CHAPTER 14 ★

LIFE IS A UNIVERSITY

One of the things I asked you to do early in this book was to look in a mirror and say hello to your competition. Everything starts and stops with you! It's *your* decision to be fit and healthy, *your* decision to get quality sleep, *your* decision how you get up in the morning, and it's *your* decision which foods enter your mouth. You are fully responsible for everything that goes on in your life. Nothing happens *to* you—it only happens *for* you.

You've discovered so much about who you are, what your purpose is, how to take control of your psychology—and, ultimately, your life. We've gone far beyond physical fitness and embraced the fact that physical fitness alone will not make you happy a person. When you combine all four elements of fitness (physical, mental, emotional, and spiritual), you have the potential not only to have a fit body but also to restructure your psychology.

The learning cannot stop here. The most successful people on this planet will tell you that life is an ongoing university. Believing in this concept means you'll have a deep dedication to making yourself your number one priority for the rest of your life. Your ongoing study is this dedication to yourself, so you can dedicate energy and vitality to your family, clients, friends, coworkers, and everyone else you love.

My North Star is all about my passion and purpose. My passion is for me, and my purpose is for others. I'm passionate about health, fitness, nutrition, business, entrepreneurship, and personal development, because I know how greatly my children, wife, business partners, trainers, and clients will benefit. My loved ones feel my purpose only when I practice my passions consistently.

THE POWER OF PROXIMITY

In addition to nutrition, you consume inputs through your eyes and ears, and those are also extremely critical. What you "take in" every day feeds your mind, body, and spirit. Inputs equal outputs. Whatever you listen to shapes your beliefs, knowledge, and behaviors. Whatever you think about the majority of the time is who you will become. Whatever you focus on is what you will believe. Inputs drive everything!

It's difficult to fix your inputs, especially when you have an emotional connection to them.

Other than yourself, the people you surround yourself with are your biggest inputs, and they are always the hardest to change. The friends we've loved for years are sometimes the biggest obstacles to overcome when creating the lasting change we desire. Don't be afraid to ditch the people who don't inspire you to grow. You'll be a reflection of the five people you hang around the most, and a crucial decision in life is figuring out your circle of influence. Misery loves company, and if your friends are miserable, they will never want to see you happy.

Even more so than friends, your parents are the biggest culprits of installing your limiting beliefs. I'm not saying don't love your parents or don't hang around them. I'm suggesting that as a grown adult, you don't have to listen to them anymore. Parents never hold you back intentionally—their lack of belief is usually their way of protecting and loving you. They don't want to see you hurt, so they put limitations around your life to help you steer clear of risk. Your parents might be wonderful, and this message might not apply to you, but surely you know someone whose parents held them back. If you do, share this book with them.

YOU DON'T NEED ANYONE ELSE'S PERMISSION TO START LIVING LIFE ON YOUR OWN TERMS.

Your friends, parents, and spouse are not the ones living your life. The days of letting them influence you in a negative way are over. Make a commitment to intentionally surround yourself with people who inspire, encourage, and motivate you to be great. This is why I created the Burn Boot Camp community—it's a second home where like-minded people can come together achieve greatness, without a single ounce of negativity.

In our time-bucket exercise, we took an inventory to gauge how much time we spent on actions that didn't align with our North Star—the inputs that needed repair. It will become plainly obvious that focusing on yourself should be top priority, once you see how it geometrically explodes other areas of your life. You'll become a leader by example for everyone you care about, including your friends and parents. Be the change you wish to see in them!

FOR ALL THE PARENTS

Being a parent completely changed my perception of what's most important in life, but it never made me question *my own* importance. I know my kids watch every move I make in my rituals, principles, and habits; they listen to my tone of voice and the way I treat my wife and friends.

I need to constantly enhance the way I communicate, handle my relationships, and grow personally, because my kids emulate everything I do.

Around the age of fifteen, kids begin to question whether or not they want to continue emulating Mom and Dad. They contemplate who they are as people and how they want to behave. My daughter is young, and she sees me work out nearly every day. She knows how to do pull-ups, push-ups, and squats. When she's fifteen, she'll decide if she still wants her gym time with Dad. I want her to see me develop and grow personally, so I can pass that on to her and empower her to live life on her own terms.

In addition to our own continual, positive development, a child's future is in the works. That means it's critical to make smart decisions about our inputs. What type of inputs are *Real Housewives*, ESPN, and other trash TV? It's garbage, and if it goes in, garbage will come out. If you constantly watch toxic programs with immature bickering, you subconsciously interpret that as an acceptable value. It's okay to consume that input as entertainment from time to time, but it can't be a ritual. Watching trash TV five nights a week for two hours straight does nothing to enhance your personal development.

Add up those two hours per day over the span of ten years, and you'll realize you have wasted months of your life.

Sure, you might be great at analyzing sports stats on ESPN, but how useful is that in the grand scheme of things? You could have used the time you wasted to write in a journal, learn a new skill, or enrich your family life. But it's not too late! Instead of watching trash TV, listen to a podcast on starting a business, or create a side hustle to maximize your financial freedom. The choice is yours.

I'm so focused on my North Star that I don't even know what TV is anymore! I only watch three major sports events: the NBA finals, the last game of the World Series, and the Super Bowl. Those are my TV "indulgences" each year. I tell you this so you know that I'm not sitting on the ground while telling you to get up and run a marathon. I practice everything in this book in my own life and have become a master of the philosophies through teaching thousands of others.

NET PERSONAL DEVELOPMENT

NET stands for "No Extra Time." This strategy for personal development maximizes each moment of your day, and you'll use every minute wisely. Life is extremely busy, and when you add kids into the mix, the perception of time is even more limited.

As I mentioned, when running in the morning, I practice active meditation by asking myself the three pregame questions: What am I grateful for? Who loves me? What are my goals for the next six to twelve months? Every minute of my time is intentionally active, and I don't spend time on anything that won't bring me closer to my goals. However, it hasn't always been this way.

When I was twenty-three, Morgan still paid my cell phone bill. The woman who had saved my life when I was young was still taking care of me as a grown-ass man, and it was embarrassing. This was so painful for me that I decided I would never be broke again, and I'd take care of her for the rest of my life. Three years later, I was a millionaire, and six years later, my companies are worth nearly $100 million. I don't tell you this to show off; I tell you this because I used to be a punk kid from Battle Creek, Michigan, who smoked weed, got drunk in high school, got beat up by his dad, and was abandoned by his mother. I decided to take control of the outcome of my life and started the process of kicking life's ass. I promise that when you are able to find a strong enough pain point in your life, you will change with a single decision, too.

I decided to give every activity I undertook a dual purpose, and by doubling the use of my time, and my life exploded! I was getting more done in a day than others were in weeks. When I needed background noise while I worked, I listened to a podcast on a revenue-generating topic. When I worked out, I didn't listen to music—I listened to motivational speakers like Mel Robbins, Jim Rohn, Gary Vaynerchuk, Ray Dalio, Tony Robbins, or Will Smith. I still practice these NET personal development activities today.

I use the tactics in this book to develop a strong psychology and to conquer my challenges and frustrations. I don't allow myself to focus on anything negative for more than five minutes, and even that has turned into about ninety seconds. I complain to my assistant, and she listens, because she knows after ninety seconds, I'll turn it into a positive and never dwell on it again.

You have to evaluate how you spend your time and be willing to make adjustments. If nothing else, build an hour into your schedule every day for NET personal development. Use that time to develop a skill that will contribute to your passion, life, and mission every single day. If you want to be successful, make your time count! If you have a demanding job, what you do from 6:00 to 10:00 p.m. every night can completely change your life! Successful people do what unsuccessful people are unwilling to do, especially when they don't feel like doing it.

★ CHAPTER 15 ★

80 PERCENT OF HAPPINESS

We've talked so much about the four areas of fitness, but now it's time to talk about one of the biggest components to happiness. Most of us spend more time with our employees, staff, or colleagues at work than we do at home. This doesn't mean work is more important than family or home life; it's simply a fact that 70 to 80 percent of our day is spent with others at work. It's no coincidence that roughly 80 percent of our happiness is connected to our mission or contribution—we spend a lot of time doing it! Any level of stress, discontent, or unease in your life is often rooted in stress from your work environment. How often do you or someone you know bring problems from work back home? The surly mood usually ends up spreading to the whole family.

When I look at issues or disagreements I've had with my wife, many have stemmed from my mood and behavior if I've had a bad day. If I had a killer day, I usually end up having a few amazing hours with my family in the evening. Early on in my career, it was hit or miss, because I wasn't mature enough to realize how important it was to be in a positive state of mind with my family, regardless of the circumstances of my day. I didn't have rituals in place, like pregaming for the day when I woke up. Stress spilled into my home life and caused arguments and discontent.

I didn't want to continue bickering at home or allowing little things to bother me, and I didn't want my mood and behavior to be the root cause. When I reflected upon why this kept happening, I finally recognized that *I* was the problem. It's difficult to embrace self-awareness and point blame at yourself for issues in your life, but it must be done. You need to properly address and resolve them, because 95 percent of the time *you* are the problem, even when you try to blame everyone else.

STRESS FRACTURES

Being an entrepreneur is demanding, and there's a fine line between what happens at home and what happens at work. I had to choose how to interpret events at work and decide where to place my focus. I learned to ask myself, "Okay, what does this mean, and how am I going to interpret it?" I found that a majority of my negativity stemmed from letting frustration and overwhelm take over. This is where the five-minute rule has worked wonders for my life.

I learned that people communicate in one of two ways: out of love, or out of a cry for help. As a business owner responsible for thousands of clients, hundreds of business partners, and hundreds of trainers, there were a lot of cries for help. I love everyone I work with, and I'm passionate about what I do, but when you lead the way for a large number of people, small hiccups are magnified. As CEO, I'm constantly dealing with the largest problems in the organization.

I used to feel overwhelmed and stressed when someone in our organization was unhappy. I pour my heart, soul, energy, and time into this mission, and I expect to be appreciated and loved no matter what. When I took a closer look, I saw that I was appreciated, but I was also expected to solve problems. What I perceived as negativity or complaining was just my personal interpretation of what people really wanted: help. Because of that, sometimes I lashed out in knee-jerk ways that were unthoughtful and unacceptable for a leader.

I have reexamined my role, and when I face problems now, I view them as opportunities. I know people appreciate me, and when I do the right things and lead the right way, they will respond in love. When I don't make the right decisions and frustration sets in, I no longer interpret that as not being appreciated. I see it as a cry for help and a lesson in improvement. Once I realized problems were merely opportunities, my life changed, and my stress was nonexistent, with no chance of spilling into my home life. I hope my example helps you prevent your work life from negatively affecting your home life. Integration of work and home is possible without sacrificing the happiness or progress of either one—you just have to take ownership if something goes wrong.

MISSION PRACTICES

In general, there are two ways to handle stress: turn the negative into a positive, or remove yourself from the situation.

If you're not happy with what you do for a living, you're not fulfilled by your mission, or you're feeling a lot of stress, it's time to look at your problems and use the negativity in a positive way. *You* choose how to focus your energy, and you can consistently move it toward a positive light. On the other hand, if you are flat out in a toxic environment that keeps you from reaching your North Star, you need to get out—and fast. Life is way too long to do something you hate doing on daily basis.

I understand there's a sense of security in earning a steady paycheck—it covers the car payment and grocery bill, but that same security can leave you paralyzed. If you dread going to work on Monday but drag yourself in because it's secure, take a moment to project that consternation over the next ten or twenty years. Considering corporate America's fickle economic state, how secure is your job? Large companies restructure all the time to increase profit margins, and you could be collateral damage.

If you're unhappy, is it because of you or your situation? If it's the situation, I recommend you get out now. Determine what you're passionate about, create a game plan, and execute. You don't want the toxicity of a poor work environment spilling over into your family life. It should be the opposite! There's no reason you can't be stoked every day at work. If you need to dedicate your evenings or get up two hours earlier to explore a new direction, do it! Ditch Netflix or the endless Facebook time, and build a side hustle from what you love.

I promise there will come a time when the effort you put in to rise to another level will outweigh your daily grind. An opportunity to transition to a new place will present itself, and you'll be ready. I've experienced this firsthand, and it's wonderful. I enjoy being a franchisor and watching my brand partners exceed what they thought possible in their careers. Many of them worked in corporate America or worked jobs they were unhappy with, and they started a

Burn Boot Camp facility on the side. Now, they are experiencing financial and emotional success!

I've been fortunate to start this successful company at a time of great innovation and creative thinking. The internet revolution is inspiring more and more people to become freelancers who work from home or grow online businesses. E-commerce is a large component of the economy, and the possibilities are limited only by your imagination and drive. Go back to that superhero moment you had as a kid. If you always wanted to be a teacher, start working toward that. Then, one day you'll stop being fine, okay, or mediocre and instead transition to being and feeling great and fulfilled. If you're a risk-taker, walk out of your job (with two weeks' notice, of course), and dive into your passion!

If you don't know what your purpose is yet, or you aren't ready to make a change, I urge you to take steps—whether slow and steady or dramatic—and use the Magic of Momentum Cycle to get you there. Progression is happiness, and that reflects on your children, family, fitness, and every other part of your life!

THE BIG PICTURE

We are looking at a holistic, global picture of your life, and we want to make it better. Many people today think success and wealth are on the same playing field—they believe success equals money and vice versa, but I can tell you from personal experience, it's not true. Don't get me wrong; money is great. I love money, and it loves me back. We have a great relationship, but it doesn't define who I am.

Money only makes you more of what you already are. If you're an asshole, money makes you a rich asshole. If you're a giving person, then you have more money to give. Money can't give you the well-rounded, peaceful feeling you get from progressing evenly in all areas of your life—the feeling of true happiness. Money will never change the way I feel about myself or the way others feel about me, but it does allow freedom.

Of course, we need money to feed our families, pay bills, and go on vacation every once in a while. However, you don't have to choose between joy and money! They are two separate things—we don't need one to have the other, but together, they enhance our quality of life. Choosing between the two is like choosing between your arm and your leg. Your leg allows you to walk and run and exercise; your arm grabs, builds, and hugs your child. If you lacked one if those limbs, your quality of life would be hindered.

Start to view money as a benefit, and build a good relationship with it. You will save it, invest it, take risks with it, and spend it. It will ebb and flow just like our motivation and demotivation to achieve our fitness goals. As long as you spend your life helping others get what they want, you will always get what *you* want in return!

★ CHAPTER 16 ★

DEVELOPING YOUR DAILY RITUALS

A *ritual* is something a person does on a consistent basis without giving it a second thought. There is no effort or practice involved once it's implemented—it's a default action. You'll find these by trial and error, experimenting with many strategies until you find a process truly enjoyable and effective. You'll start using strategies, and then pivot. You might stop using one, two, or four of them; take what you learned from each one, and figure out what's best for you.

The Perfect Day isn't a myth or some unattainable fantasy. This is a real, long-term goal that requires you to work backwards in your life to determine the action you must take today. This is your passion and meaning—this is what you desire for *you*. Your North Star is your purpose and *why* you want to achieve your Perfect Day. Your rituals are the building blocks to ultimately architect the skyscraper of your dreams. Or, in other words, they are your strategy to build fulfillment.

Many people see rituals as habits, but they are two very different things. A habit is something you do, or should do. A ritual is something you *must* do—it's done on a daily basis to fulfill our needs as human beings and create progression toward happiness.

Habits tend to appear without conscious effort, like texting while driving (please don't do that) or mindless eating. Rituals, on the other hand, are things you make a focused effort to do, and you've determined you must do them to maintain happiness.

Habits will fluctuate; rituals are a way of living. Rituals create discipline, and discipline is like a muscle. The more you flex and work your discipline muscle, the stronger it will be, and the more confidence you will develop. There will be things in your life you must do, that you won't feel like doing, but remember: successful people *always* do what's necessary—their North Star powerfully pulls them toward their goals. Just as you have to practice push-ups to get better at them, you have to practice discipline to get better at it. Discipline is the key to creating and maintaining rituals, and then making them default actions.

The constant practice of discipline will give you the strength to say "no" to all that doesn't align with your North Star. And when you slip up (and you will), you won't beat yourself up. You'll use it as an opportunity to learn.

We've created expansive opportunity for you. We've deleted old, outdated psychology and installed a brand-new way of thinking. We've not once closed off your options. Doesn't it feel good to know that failure is part of the process? The only thing you must fear in this life is regret. So, let's take this new mindset and create a plan. Let's begin designing your life!

EIGHT DAILY RITUALS: PLAN DESIGN

I want you to answer the questions below for each of the eight daily rituals, and then design your *own* plan. It may be necessary to flip back to previous chapters and take a second look at the options I've laid out. I highly suggest getting an accountability partner—maybe someone you've purchased this book for—and build your plans together!

★ **Pregaming:** These are the things you do right when you wake up. What will you do first thing in the morning? What habits are you going to change? What rituals will you adopt? How will you spend your first ten to fifteen minutes of the day?

★ **Nutrition:** What types of foods will you eat? How will

you resist temptation? What's your ritual for travel or vacation? What other strategies will you use to ensure you are maximizing your energy? How will you stay balanced?

★ **Fitness:** How will you make time for exercise? What time of the day will you work out? When will you schedule your workouts? How often will you train? What commitment will you make to practice fitness, even when you don't feel like it?

★ **Family:** When will you designate family time? How will you integrate family, work, and yourself? How will you better connect with your spouse? If you have kids, what commitment will you make to them? Which friends deserve to be around you, and which ones don't?

★ **Personal Development:** How many hours per day are you committed to growing personally? How will you use NET personal development? What inputs do you need to absorb? What inputs do you need to get rid of? Who will you hang around on a daily basis? What does your ongoing university look like?

★ **Connection:** How will you connect more closely with your higher power? What commitment are you willing to make to enhance your spiritual fitness? When will you make time to connect spiritually?

★ **Mission:** How will you gain more financial freedom? How will you increase your impact on the world? What will you do to create more fulfillment in your work? If you dislike your job, what steps will you take daily to find something you're passionate about?

* **Bedtime:** How will you prepare for the next day before you go to bed? What commitment are you willing to make to sleep peacefully? How much sleep are you committed to getting to optimize your energy? What will you do to ensure you are getting REM sleep?

All of these rituals combined can create happiness. You have to make daily deposits into each one and minimize withdrawals. If any ritual falls into the red, that means trouble. A wildly successful career is great, but if your family life suffers because of it, you need to show your family some love. If your fitness level drops because you spend every waking moment with your family, you need to add fitness into the mix. Happiness is about *full integration* of these eight areas. You don't need to have all the answers right now. If this is too much to do all at once, I suggest starting with the most difficult one first. Always remember that progression equals happiness, and changing even one element can drastically impact your happiness.

TRANSFORMATIVE LANGUAGE MEETS RITUALS

Have you ever heard the phrase, "I fell off the wagon over the holidays?" Talk about transformative language! I usually challenge anyone who says this to show me their bruises and the busted wagon. This makes them laugh and breaks their pattern.

Every month of the year has a holiday or event loaded with temptation. Right off the bat, there are New Year's Eve and New Year's Day, with food everywhere. Valentine's Day is filled with candy. Somebody's birthday comes along, and there's cake. Summer is barbeque and beer season. Fall is apple-orchard time. Then it's Halloween, Thanksgiving, and Christmas. There's always an opportunity to load up on too much food or too many holiday desserts, and there are times when you will travel away from your rituals. But don't let those ten or fifteen days dictate what the rest of the year looks like.

If you take a break from your rituals, don't convince yourself you "fell off the wagon." Understand it's only a temporary deviation from your healthy path. Be confident, and return to the rituals you've created. Trade expectation for appreciation, and be prepared to face temptation around every corner. It's okay to give in sometimes—as long as you consistently make choices that move you toward your North Star.

CONCLUSION

TAKING MASSIVE ACTION

You've learned a lot in this book! Every chapter gave you tools and opportunities to decide whether or not to shift your mindset. I want it for you, but *you* have to want it more.

None of this matters if you don't take action right now—and not just any action, *massive* action. Remember, knowledge is not power; it's *potential* power. Without action, knowledge is nothing. You've spent precious hours of your life reading this book, learning ways to better yourself and to get to the next level. It's time to follow through!

I want you to stop right now and do something, or schedule something that will help get you to your North Star. Ignorance is not bliss. You cannot ignore the fact that if it's not on your schedule, it's not going to happen. Don't allow ignorance to push you backward.

IGNORANCE IN YOUR PROFESSIONAL LIFE LEADS TO POVERTY. IGNORANCE IN YOUR FAMILY LIFE LEADS TO DIVORCE. IN FITNESS, IT'S A BODY WITHOUT ENERGY.

Without pregaming your day, ignorance is a mind riddled with negativity.

If you implement just one strategy given in this book, you can drastically change your life. Look at the areas that need consistent attention, consider the eight rituals, and then determine which ones are in the black and which are in the red. Which ones need a deposit? Which ones are you focusing on too much? Is your focus hurting other areas in your life? Are you trying to balance your life, rather than integrate it?

Creating lasting change can be hard to do on your own. Oftentimes, you may feel like you're on an island with no one to talk to. Maybe your friends and family don't understand the changes you've made since you've learned that happiness is in your control.

I started the Burn Boot Camp community because so many people want to be healthy, but preconditioning and their current reality hold them back from realizing their true potential. They needed to enter an environment where they could be successful—a place that empowered them to make choices for their own lives, on their own terms. I've created an entire movement that builds people up rather than breaking them down. Being part of a community allows each person to flourish, and everything we do aligns with the philosophies and principles to achieve ultimate happiness.

If you have negative people in your life and you need a community, we're here for you! There are Burn Boot Camps all across the country, with many ways to connect. You can meet other people who want to better their lives alongside you. There's always conversation on our social media pages and informational podcasts, and you can connect directly with me as well. I spend an hour every night engaging with people and their goals. If you want to rise to yet another level, you're not alone!

I genuinely hope you've enjoyed this process of bettering yourself. I also hope that you recall these principles often and use them to improve your life. I encourage you to take action right now. Don't wait until tomorrow! I would enjoy hearing from you and hearing how this book helped change your life.

You're not alone in this journey. I'm here as a mentor and

leader, and to help you grow. After reading this book, take a picture and post it to Instagram or Facebook and let me know how it's helped you in your life! If you or anyone in your life needs help in any of these areas, I can help you. This world has too much negativity, and together, we are creating a revolution of happiness through the gateway of fitness!

Join me on my Private Facebook Page along with others who desire to stop starting over. Search "Stop Starting Over with Devan Kline" and request to be added to the group.

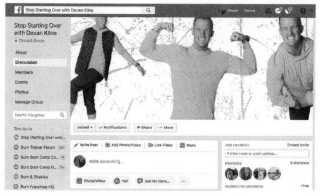

Join my Facebook group: devankline.com/fbgroup

 Follow along on Instagram: instagram.com/devan.kline

 Subscribe to my Youtube Channel: youtube.com/DevanKlineFitness

 Read my articles on my blog: devankline.com/blog

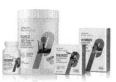

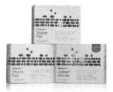

Afterburn
devankline.com/afterburn

Shaklee Fitness Pack
devankline.com/fitpack

Shaklee Vitalizer
devankline.com/vitalizer

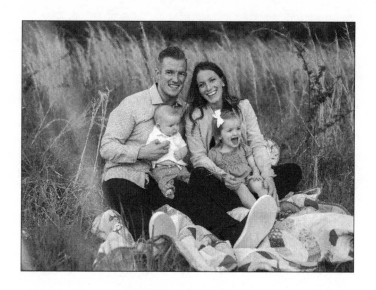

ABOUT THE AUTHOR

DEVAN KLINE and his wife, Morgan, are cofounders of Burn Boot Camp, a fitness empire they started in a parking lot at twenty-four years old. Devan integrates a revolutionary approach to physical, mental, emotional, and spiritual health that is changing the world. Burn Boot Camp already serves hundreds of locations, with plans to open thousands of locations globally over the coming years. The Klines reside in Cornelius, North Carolina, with their daughter, son, and two German shepherds.